Angela Ardalis-Holt

BEYOND YOUR NUMBERS

Connect the Pieces
to a Path of
Amazing Health

ANGELA ANDALCIO-HOLTZ

BEYOND YOUR NUMBERS
Connect the Pieces to a Path of Amazing Health

Copyright © 2018 by Angela Andalcio-Holtz

The content of this book is for general instruction only. Each person's physical, emotional, and spiritual condition is unique. The instruction in this book is not intended to replace or interrupt the reader's relationship with a physician or other professional. Please consult your doctor for matters pertaining to your specific health and diet.

No part of this publication may be reproduced, distributed, or transmitted in any form or by any means, including photocopying, recording, or other electronic or mechanical methods, without the prior written permission of the publisher or author, except in the case of brief quotations embodied in critical reviews and certain other noncommercial uses permitted by copyright law. All rights reserved. For permission r equests, contact author and publisher: angela@myuniquepathway.com.

To contact the author, visit: myuniquepathway.com

ISBN 978-0-9994823-1-5

Printed in the United States of America

Acknowledgements

I extend my deepest gratitude to my daughter Rachelle. Her patience, endless literary advice, and overall guidance were crucial in the making of this book. I want to thank my son, Ryan, for the computer tips and my daughter Aundrea for her thoughtful, health-probing enquiries. I also thank my daughter-in-law Ali for her input that helped me to broaden the scope of my book.

I am grateful to my brother Herman, who encouraged me with his many inspiring life stories and tactful criticisms. I acknowledge my former husband, Bob, for sharing the book *Integrative Nutrition: Feed Your Hunger for Health & Happiness*, which introduced me to the nontraditional school of nutrition, the Institute for Integrative Nutrition® (IIN®).

I would like to give a special thanks to Joshua Rosenthal, founder of IIN®, and his diverse and knowledgeable staff. Along with Lillian Munt (a former professor from 2002), they served as the water and sunshine to nurture the seed planted in me to write this book.

Finally, I would like to recognize my friends Ian and Mike for sharing some of their unbiased perspectives and Dr. Barrett for his concrete and scientific evaluation.

Dedication

I dedicate this book to my children Rachelle, Ryan, Aundrea, and their spouses—your love and support have made me learn to appreciate life to its fullest and to live in the moment. To my grandchildren Enya, Jaden, Rylie, and Evan—you light up my life.

To the readers, ready and committed to connect the pieces—High Five!

Contents

Introduction	11
1 - Amazing Health—Your Score	13
2 - Know Your Numbers	25
3 - Nutrition Overview — Armor for Your Health	43
4 - Metabolism and Sustained Energy	75
5 - Another Type of Nourishment	83
6 - Creating Your Unique Plate	93
7 - Cook Once, Eat Three Times or More	103
8 - Connect the Pieces	109
Recipes - Let's Start Cooking	113
Helpful Websites	125
References	127

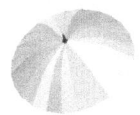

Introduction

When I had first thought about writing this book, I asked myself what would make my perspective on this topic different from other health and wellness authors. As a medical technologist I have been a witness to the alarming increase in dangerously unhealthy lab numbers (glucose, triglycerides, hemoglobin, etc.) for over two decades. These "critical lab results" (originating from the performance of several analyzers and the use of the microscope) are the numbers often associated with diseases such as diabetes, heart problems, cancer, stroke, and many other metabolic abnormalities. As an Institute for Integrative Nutrition® (IIN®) certified health coach, I am bewildered because I know most of these critical lab results can be avoided when we take responsibility for our health.

This book will explain how and why simple lifestyle changes can make a difference in preventing certain diseases. Studies have proven time and time again that achieving amazing health involves several aspects of your life—consuming the correct foods, participating in regular physical activity, and forming a support system for life's challenges. You might be surprised to discover certain events in your life nourish you also. You may feel and look fit, but how do you know if your overall lifestyle is supporting and maintaining your nutritional status? In this book, I will share health measures to protect you against many preventable diseases. This includes an overview of nutrition and exercise, a standard wellness screen, and the numbers on which to focus. I will also share with you a non-typical laboratory test that goes to the cellular level to disclose if subtle nutritional deficiencies are sabotaging your health. If you are new to cooking, you will find a few basic recipes in the Recipe section that can be easily modified to create meal variations.

Remember, it is never too late to get on a healthy path. These concepts of health are available for you to insert into your lifestyle to achieve your health goals beyond your numbers.

Whether you've given up, need a stronger nudge in the right direction, or feel "too old for that", my aim is to inspire you to achieve the best "you" you can be. Only you can be in control of your personal health and committing to do so should be your number one goal.

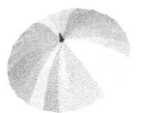

1

Amazing Health—Your Score

*"You have brains in your head. You have feet in your shoes.
You can steer yourself any direction you choose."*
-Dr. Seuss[1]

What is your definition of amazing health? Is it being physically fit? Is it being able to fight off the common cold? How about living independently through your senior years? I believe it's all of this and more.

Have you ever sat down to piece together a jigsaw puzzle with the completed image on the cover of the box in front of you? The real challenge and reward is putting it all together to achieve that very image. Attaining and maintaining a healthy status can be compared to connecting the pieces of a jigsaw puzzle. These individual pieces come from many aspects of your life: **nutrition, physical activity, emotional well-being and preventive health actions.** Fitting together these aspects of your life so that you can enjoy amazing health is well within your grasp. However, you need to first understand how these four major pieces fit together. Each of these health pieces include features that work together to produce *your umbrella of protection on a path to amazing health.* As you connect these four aspects of your life, they will become the foundation for maintaining your amazing health and creating your personal anti-aging habits. Only you can discover how to connect these pieces to your life as *you take responsibility for your health and act accordingly.*

Nutrition

Nutrition is a major piece to this puzzle and comes directly from the foods you eat. It fuels your body and its systems with the energy and nutrients needed for growth, repair, and reproduction. Because each of us is genetically and biochemically unique, my body's nutritional requirements will be different from what your body requires. For example, there might be some foods that you enjoy but discover early or later in life that they should be avoided because of allergic reactions. These same foods may work well for others and vice versa. Researchers now include nutritional genomics in the discussion of optimal health. Nutritional genomics is a scientific field that explores the interaction of nutrition, genes, and environmental factors coming together to impact your overall immunity.[2]

You might be wondering, "if genes determine certain health risks, how can diet prevent those threats?" Certain genetic changes can be either inherited or acquired throughout life. Nutrients found in foods and the functioning of a strong immune system can protect the DNA that control cell growth from damages and mutations. It has been shown that some types of mutations or genetic damage can increase the risks for certain diseases (e.g., cancer.) Therefore, **you need to know which foods serve you best.** In addition to eating these foods, quality supplements can help you get the optimal amounts of nutrients necessary to sustain a healthy life.[3]

Physical Activity

Maintaining physical activity is another major piece to your health puzzle. I emphasize it is **extremely important** to engage in daily activity that will utilize most of your muscles. You don't have to join a gym to get active. Household chores, on-the-job activity, dog – walking, or any type of regular movements is a good start. Having a gym membership can only enhance your everyday activity level. However, your gym membership, like any activity program you choose to do, is only beneficial if you use it. Regular activity helps maintain a healthy body, mind, and weight, unique to your age, height, gender, and genetic makeup.

Emotional Well-Being

Another significant piece to your health puzzle is safeguarding and nourishing your emotional and mental health (i.e., your emotional well-being). This nourishment derives from your initiatives and experiences gained through your social, spiritual, intellectual, environmental, and occupational happenings, as you progress through your life.[4] Positive outcomes provide a gratifying energy like no other, but negative outcomes can be devastating. If support and guidance are not pursued to stabilize your mental health, the effects of negative energy can be long lasting.

Preventive Health Actions

The final major piece to your health puzzle is preventive health actions. This includes annual physical and wellness screens that provide numbers that—when monitored and understood—shed a light on your health status. Dental checkups twice a year are important; and as you approach middle age, comprehensive visual and auditory examinations should be included. These preventive health actions are needed to configure this piece into your health puzzle.

Knowledge is crucial. If you don't have a broad view of how to fit these essential components into your health plan, you can unknowingly compromise your natural suit of armor—your immune system—and become a prime target for multiple attacks on your health. These attacks can come in the form of **heart disease, stroke, cardiovascular diseases,** *metabolic syndrome, gum disease, cancer, and other diseases.* Having this knowledge and *implementing it* will also serve as a positive example for your children and other family members to replicate.

Your Natural Suit of Armor

Whether you wake up eager and ready to take on the day or you are still exhausted from caring for your family or working at the job, it's important to understand that your body is constantly operating behind the scenes to achieve a healthy balance. This balance is maintained by **seven remarkable body systems.** They are your immune, digestive, circulatory, nervous, endocrine, musculature, and skeletal systems. To sustain their functions, **each body system needs adequate levels of micronutrients (vitamin C, Selenium, etc.) and macronutrients (protein, carbohydrates, etc.)** that come from specific foods and supplements. Of all the body systems, the immune system is your defense shield and is directly associated with the prevention of disease and protecting your health. The immune system is like a suit of armor protecting you. This system relies on many other unique defense mechanisms built into the rest of your body's systems.[5] You might be surprised to learn that most of the cells involved in the immune system reside in your gut. This is where trillions of specific microbes are found performing a task unique only to them and are referred to as your microbiota. They increase your ability to metabolize foods with enzymes only they can provide.[6]

Your immune system plays a substantial role in the healing processes such as repairing skin abrasions and fighting off certain bacteria, viruses, and parasites. This healing process begins with a complex internal development called inflammation. Each time you find yourself dealing with bruised skin, a sprained ankle, or the common cold, your body reacts to protect and heal itself with inflammation, termed **Acute inflammation.**[7]

You may notice redness, swelling and pain, and a rise in body temperature as your body is responding with the release of several chemical messengers, all with the single goal to help the body return to a healthy state. Once that healthy state has been achieved, the inflammation subsides. However, an ongoing inflammation status may develop that can cause serious damage over time. This might be activated by underlying infection, consuming certain processed foods, allergies, or irritations caused by other factors (i.e., environmental). This inflammation is termed **Chronic inflammation**. Research has shown that many serious diseases, including heart disease and some cancers, are fueled by inflammation.[8]

The suffix-*itis* indicates inflammation in medical terminology. For example, arthritis is inflammation of the joints, periodontitis is inflammation of the gums, and appendicitis is inflammation of the appendix. It has been seen that inflammation in one part of the body can cause repercussions to develop in other areas (often distant and in otherwise unrelated parts of the body). The immune system also helps to eliminate potentially toxic molecules that can generate **Oxidative Stress** during the normal processes of metabolism. These molecules are sometimes referred to as **Free Radicals** or **Reactive Oxygen Species** (because of their chemical structure).[9] Free radicals can also be derived from the detoxification of pollutants and other harmful components of biological structures within the body. Some of the molecular structures may have originated from carcinogens absorbed from the air, water, or even from some foods (farmed with pesticides). Micronutrients from specific foods and in the required amounts, are the ammunition used by your immune system to help remove, neutralize, and regulate free radicals. (See Chapter 3).

Your suit of armor prevails when the major health puzzle pieces are in place and working in synergy at an optimum level. *You may not be able to escape all the attacks from illnesses, but the stronger your immune system, the faster your body will recover from attacks or surgical procedures—enabling your return to a stable state.*

Some Avoidable Statistics

If you're like most people, (myself included), the closer to home a tragedy occurs, the greater the effect is on you. Now, think about your circle of friends and family. Can you name one person in your life that has been affected by a preventable disease? According to the American Heart Association, (AHA), one out of seven people in your circle may die of a cardiovascular disease.[10] Cardiovascular disease is the leading global cause of death. Each year, about 550,000 people in the United States have a heart attack for the first time and almost half of those people will have a recurrent attack.[11] Globally, 17.3 million people die every year from cardiovascular disease, and that number is expected to grow to more than 23.6 million by 2030.[12] In the United States alone, over 2,000 people die each day from a heart attack; that's one every 40 seconds![13]

Did you know that stroke is the single most preventable disease as well as the number one cause of disability? It is also the fifth most frequent cause of death in the United States, killing nearly 129,000 people every year.[14] The brain, along with the spinal cord and nerves, receives, processes, and relays information to and from different parts of your body and from your environment. Just like when your computer short circuits or crashes and can no longer perform, when a stroke occurs, the brain may "crash" if it is deprived of oxygen.

Both direct and indirect costs of cardiovascular diseases and stroke total more than $316.6 billion.[15] This cost impacts the nation, your employer, insurance companies, your pocket book, and **ultimately your quality of life.**

AHA lists **seven key risk factors and behaviors that automatically put you at increased danger for developing cardiovascular disease and stroke.** They are smoking, physical inactivity, low-nutrient diet, abnormal lipid levels (fat present in the blood), high blood pressure, elevated blood glucose or diabetes, and being overweight or obese. When three or more of these risk factors occur together, their combined effects contribute to an even greater risk for heart disease and stroke.[16] Can you identify any of these risk factors in your own life? When was your last wellness screen done, and do you recall your numbers?

Another major health concern on the rise is ***metabolic syndrome*** and it is diagnosed when a combination of three or more of the following risk factors are seen together: high blood pressure, increased abdominal body fat, elevated blood glucose, and abnormal lab results for lipid levels.[17] Metabolic syndrome has become a major health concern for the Western world and I would be doing you a great disservice if I didn't talk to you at least briefly about it. It is reported that almost 23% of American adults are afflicted with Metabolic Syndrome.[18] Some of the independent risk factors that lead to heart disease, diabetes, and stroke, mentioned above, when combined, can lead to metabolic syndrome. Can you see how this health threat is just as preventable as diabetes, heart disease, and stroke? Most of the health risks associated with metabolic syndrome have no overt symptoms, except there might be a bulging waistline or, if your blood sugar is elevated, you may experience increased urination, thirst, fatigue, and even blurred vision—the first signs of diabetes. Weight gain can be subtle as it goes relatively unnoticed when it occurs slowly over the course of many years making it appear normal to you. Other times, weight gain happens quickly and becomes alarmingly obvious. Whether it occurs slowly or rapidly, this unnecessary weight gain can inadvertently catapult you towards some of the preventable diseases mentioned in this book. Without a wellness screen to confirm these symptoms, you may not even be aware that you have this syndrome. If you can avoid falling prey to this syndrome, you will be well on your way to enriching your health. If you happen to be diagnosed with metabolic syndrome or any of its risk factors, it is not necessarily a death sentence. With ***persistent modifications*** in your diet and lifestyle and collaboration with your primary care doctor, you can return to a healthy status.

According to AHA, keeping track of the following risk factors, modifying your lifestyle and behaviors when necessary, can prevent you from becoming a statistic.[19]

- **Smoking:** If you are a smoker you are at risk of developing certain cancers. This is because cigarette smoke, like other pollutants in the air (e.g., paint and exhaust fumes) can damage a cell's DNA, which is the controlling factor for normal growth and function within the body. When the DNA is damaged, it creates a weakened immune system that becomes overwhelmed by other attackers.[20]

- **Diet:** Avoid regularly consuming foods and drinks high in caloric density (e.g., beverages sweetened with more than two teaspoons of sugar, sweet rolls and cakes) with little or no nutrient value. They promote weight gain and cause nutritional deficiencies that eventually offset the functions of organs in the body systems.

- **Physical Inactivity:** Avoid a sedentary lifestyle. Little or no daily physical activity can lead to obesity and a decline in your overall health—*exercise is essential.*

- **Genetic Inheritance:** You can thank Mom and Dad for this one. If you have a family history of type 2 diabetes **OR** you're a female with a history of diabetes during pregnancy (gestational diabetes), you are at a greater risk of developing diabetes after your pregnancy is over. Also, babies born of mothers with gestational diabetes are more likely to develop type 2 diabetes later in life.[21] Be very vigilant with your lifestyle if this applies to you.

- **Ethnicity:** Certain ethnic groups show a higher risk for developing type 2 diabetes. These groups include African American, Hispanic American, Native American, and Asian American.[22] Despite the statistics that show certain American ethnic groups are more susceptible to type 2 diabetes, anyone who is not proactive with diet and lifestyle habits can be at risk.

- **Age:** With the aging process the immune system declines, which makes you more susceptible to diseases.[23] Therefore, it will benefit you to develop healthy habits (as mentioned in this book) as early as possible to maintain a strong immune system to experience amazing health.

A physical and wellness screen can reveal if any of the above-mentioned preventable conditions are surfacing. If you have already been diagnosed with any of the above risk factors; are on medication for diabetes, high blood pressure (hypertension), or abnormal lipids; or suffer from any other chronic illnesses such as arthritis, fatigue, or cardiovascular disease, a return to a healthy status is possible using some of the information in this book while partnering with your primary care doctor. The ***key is consistently following a plan to make improvements.*** When you strive to maintain a healthy lifestyle, not only will this action benefit you, but it will have a positive influence on your family, friends, and coworkers.

Your Score

You might be currently experiencing challenging blocks impeding your ability to achieve healthy goals you have set for yourself. Reflecting on what we have gone over, take the time now to evaluate your current health status, habits, and behaviors with this short quiz to see where you are on your current health path. This exercise serves to create awareness of some of your habits and is by no means the only solution to managing your health status.

1. Do you have annual physicals, including dental checkups? _____

    Yes = 10 points   No = 0 point

2. Do you include five or more vegetables and fruits in most meals each day?_____

   Yes = 10 points   No = 0 points

3. How many times per week are you physically active for at least 25 minutes? _____

   5 times per week = 10 points   3 times per week = 5 points
   None = 0 points

4. Do you have a plan in place to deal with stress?_____

   Yes = 10 points   No = 0 points

5. Are you a smoker?_____

   No = 10 points   Yes = 0 points

What Is Your Score? _____

50 Great job—you are connecting the pieces and heading in the right direction!

40–45 Nice work. However, you may need to add more to your healthy habits.

30–40 This is the time to make some improvements to your lifestyle.

Less than 30. Now is the time to reconsider your current health and lifestyle habits; connect the health pieces to make significant changes.

Planning Preventive Health Measures

Wouldn't it be perfect if there was an audible alarm in your body that could alert you when things are being disrupted—one like the beeping alarms in several laboratory analyzers that alert technologists to the need for immediate attention? We do have innate alarm warnings, just not as loud. Persistent occurrences such as weight loss or weight gain, digestive distress (this can be loud at times), lingering mental stress and fatigue, allergic responses (if recognized as such), and other feelings of pain and discomfort are the many signals that are inaudible yet serve as alarms to warn us of disrupting or impending malfunctions. So, too, are lingering abnormal lab numbers. Wellness laboratory screens can provide vital information on your general health and can indicate the possible beginning of a disease.

When any of these alarms "sound," you need to take a moment to ponder what foods you are eating, or have not been eating, and what has changed in your life such as your environment, occupation, or social interactions. This approach may appear simple, but it can lead to distinctive answers that can be helpful to your doctor, also.

The body is remarkable and resilient. It was designed to heal itself, but you need to encourage the process and at the same time plan for emergency situations. You need to prepare and have access to medical and wellness professionals so that you can get the appropriate medical care and treatment when needed. This can make a difference to your recovery and health maintenance.

Getting Started

If you have individual health insurance or are insured through your employer but haven't selected a primary care doctor, start the process to select one. Your primary care doctor should be one with whom you feel comfortable discussing not only your health issues, but also some of your life experiences. Referrals can be found from family members, friends, colleagues, and your healthcare plan (depending on the flexibility of your healthcare plan). If you do not currently have health insurance, you can ask your local health authorities for assistance. Many agencies are available to help, such as your local city, county, or township office. Once you find a primary care doctor and schedule your first visit, be prepared to fill out medical history forms. These forms will ask questions about your current health and any health issues you've had in the past. Prior to your first visit, it's a good idea to talk with your senior family members who might have had health issues in the past or are currently dealing with health problems. A family history of heart disease, diabetes, or cancer can increase your risk of developing similar diseases as mentioned above. However, with a practical, preventive approach, you can postpone, avoid, or reverse some of these vulnerable conditions.[24]

Write down your acquired information and any allergies you are aware of as well as any medications, vitamins, or supplements you currently take. Finally, jot down questions you have for your doctor to address any personal health concerns. Bring all of this with you on your first visit and don't be afraid to reference this information when you are with your doctor. Thorough documentation will help your doctor to better understand your health care needs and help to build a relationship so that he or she can point you in the right direction. Be truthful and don't leave anything out even if you think it is trivial.

You also need to visit a dentist for oral checkups every six months. Studies have shown gum disease, with the underlying factor of inflammation, puts you at greater risk for developing heart disease and other health related problems. This preventive action can even protect against oral cancer.[25]

As you approach middle age, yearly comprehensive visual and auditory examinations can be a valuable health measure to allow early discovery of diminishing sight and hearing. Science provides many corrective tools to help compensate for deficiencies in these areas and utilizing them (when required) will allow you to continue living a productive lifestyle as you enter your golden years.

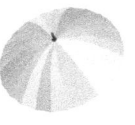

2

Know Your Numbers

Annual physical and wellness screens are important steps in becoming proactive with your health. They will provide vital information about your general health and can indicate the possible beginning of a disease, which is crucial in fighting and overcoming it. The numbers resulting from your physical exam and laboratory tests help you gauge and monitor your health status.

One of the questions I always ask during a health coaching interview is, "What was your last blood glucose number?" Most of the time, this number cannot be recalled, and the health connection is not recognized. How about you? Can you recall your most recent blood glucose number or your last blood pressure numbers? Have you ever discussed your body mass index (BMI) number with your doctor? Do you pay attention to your triglyceride and high-density lipid (HDL) numbers? The results from these measurements are the numbers that will influence your course of actions as you focus on improving or maintaining your health. These are a few of the numbers I want you to remember because they will indicate if you are at risk for developing the diseases mentioned earlier, ***including metabolic syndrome.*** (These tests and numbers will be preceded by the @ symbol).

Most primary care doctors offer a wellness screen that is age and gender appropriate. At your annual physical and wellness screen, your doctor may first complete some of the following assessments and then order laboratory testing for a different time:

- Blood pressure
- Body temperature
- Pulse rate
- Respiratory rate
- Height and weight (to calculate your BMI)
- Skin exam

In addition to the above evaluations women may also receive a pelvic exam, pap test and breast exam. Women over 50, may receive interval screens such as a mammogram, bone mineral density test, and a colonoscopy. Depending on health history, the interval screens might be suggested at an earlier age.[26]

Men, over the age of 50, or depending on health history, may receive the assessments mentioned above plus a digital prostate examination and a colonoscopy.[27]

Let's take a closer look at some of the numbers to remember and why they are important.

@ Blood Pressure Numbers

According to the Center for Disease Control, high blood pressure is called the "silent killer" because often there are no signs or symptoms.[28] You may not know your blood pressure is high or out of your specific healthy range until a measurement is taken. Two separate numbers are recorded when the measurement is taken. The higher number is referred to as the systolic blood pressure, shown when the heart muscle contracts. The lower number is referred to as the diastolic blood pressure, shown when the heart muscle relaxes. Both systolic and diastolic pressure are recorded as millimeters of mercury. If the measurement reads 120 systolic and 80 diastolic, you would say "120 over 80" or write 120/80 mm Hg. A blood pressure that is equal to or less than 120/80 mm Hg is considered normal. A blood pressure of 140/90 mm Hg or greater is considered high. Each 20/10 mm Hg increment over 115/75 doubles the risk of heart attack (coronary heart disease), heart failure, brain attack (stroke), and kidney disease in individuals between the ages of 40 and 70. Life Extension, (an integrated, scientific and wide-ranging health establishment) promotes a blood pressure of 115/75 mm Hg as an optimal target to achieve the most health benefits.[29]

@ BMI/Waist Circumference Numbers

Have you ever paid attention to the numbers for your body mass index (BMI) and waist circumference? Measurements of your height and weight are used in a mathematical formula to assess how much fat is in your body. The derived number is referred to as BMI and can be a good gauge of your risk for diseases that include hypertension (high blood pressure), type 2 diabetes, heart disease, and some forms of cancer. According to American Institute for Cancer Research (AICR), "Excess body fat is a cause of a number of chronic diseases."[30]

Here is the formula to calculate your BMI:[31]
   (weight * 703) / height^2
   (Weight refers to pounds, and height refers to inches)

For example, if you weigh 225 pounds and you are 6 feet 2 inches (or 74 inches) tall, this is how you would calculate your BMI:

BMI = (225 * 703) / (74 * 74)
BMI = (158,175) / (5,476)
BMI = 28.9

BMI Ranges

30.0 or Higher	Obese
25.0 to 29.9	Overweight
18.5 to 24.9	Normal
Less than 18.5	Underweight

(Note that there are some circumstances for which the results of this formula may not apply such as professional athletes or weight lifters, manual workers, due to their muscle to fat ratio).[32]

Waist Circumference Numbers

Your BMI may fall into an acceptable range; however, abdominal fat can still be a culprit. You should be concerned if your waist circumference is greater than 40 inches (men) or greater than 35 inches (women).[33]

Clinical Laboratory Numbers

A laboratory test is a procedure in which a sample of blood, urine, body fluid, or tissue is examined to get information about a person's general health or to probe further into a suspicious health condition. This method of clinical investigation plays a major role in modern medicine which helps with diagnosis and screening of many health situations. Most standard lab tests give a snapshot of a person's current health status.

The interpretation and function of laboratory tests involve numbers that include reference ranges. The reference range can be considered the ideal range your test result should fall within to be considered "normal." This range is usually listed alongside your lab results with a low-end number and a high-end number. For example, if your fasting glucose test result is 80 mg/dL (milligrams per deciliter), then the format may read:

Fasting Glucose	Reference Range
80 mg/dL	75 to 99 mg/dL

So, how are reference ranges set and who determines what's "normal?" The manufacturers of laboratory instruments determine the reference ranges by using statistical data obtained after testing large numbers of healthy individuals of varying age and gender without clinical disease. These reference ranges can differ to some extent depending on the population and the geographical location that the laboratory is serving. What is then selected as the "normal" reference ranges for a clinical laboratory will be represented after an adjustment is made for the population being served. If your test results fall outside the reference range, it can be an indication of an underlying imbalance that may require further testing to find the root cause. However, there is no single reference range that applies to everyone. Close to or within the recommended range may be a specific number unique to your genetic makeup that works best for you. You will discover this number as time goes on. You can use reference ranges to attain your personal optimal numbers as one of your goals.[34]

Preanalytical Factors that May Affect Your Numbers

Many preanalytical factors can affect your numbers however, here are some important issues on which to begin focusing.[35]

Fasting

Some tests require a fast (no consumption of food) for 12 hours before blood is collected. This is usually recommended for glucose and lipid testing to assess if the breakdown and assimilation of nutrients into cells are normal and not hindered by any malfunction of organs. If you do not fast for the appropriate time prior to your scheduled tests, your numbers are highly prone to be inaccurate and may require you redo this test.

Medications

Some medications and multivitamins can interfere with certain tests, causing false positive or false negative results. Be aware if this applies to you.

Exercise

Your body releases certain biochemicals when you exercise; therefore, exercising before specific lab tests can cause false results.

Pregnancy

Hormonal changes during pregnancy can skew results.

Dehydration

When your body is dehydrated, the blood can become more concentrated and can cause false elevated results.

Laboratory Wellness Tests/Screens

Here is a list of traditional wellness tests for you to keep in mind and to use to start a conversation with your primary care doctor. I will elaborate on some of these tests so that you can understand the connection to the body and what their numbers/results could reveal. The labs requested for your wellness tests may read like this:

Comprehensive Metabolic Profile (CMP)

Lipid Profile

Hemoglobin (Hgb) or Complete Blood Count (CBC)

Vitamin D

Glycated Hemoglobin (A1C or hemoglobin A1C, depending on age and health history)

The number of tests included in a wellness screen can be overwhelming. However, becoming familiar with some of these tests *(preceded with the @ symbol)* will be useful as you monitor your health. Keep in mind that these screens are all used to identify if you are at risk for several diseases including diabetes, heart problems, metabolic syndrome, or cancer and give a snapshot of general well-being. These tests should be included in your wellness screens because abnormal results can be "red flags" for several health issues as mentioned above.

Comprehensive Metabolic Profile (CMP)

This is a group of tests that reflects a general status of organ function and some levels of blood components; they include:

Fasting blood glucose, AST (SGOT), ALT (SGPT), LDH, total bilirubin, alkaline phosphatase, BUN, creatinine, BUN/creatinine ratio, uric acid, total protein, albumin, globulin, albumin/globulin ratio, calcium, sodium, potassium, phosphorus, iron, and chloride.[36]

@Fasting Blood Glucose

Glucose measurements are used to detect diabetes and evaluate a range of other carbohydrate metabolic disorders. Glucose is derived from the breakdown of food-carbohydrates, one of the body's fuel supplies. The pancreas produces insulin that is responsible for the entry of glucose into the cells of your body. This test requires a 12 hour fast before blood is taken. If food is eaten within that fasting time, glucose levels may be elevated.

Glucose Reference Range:
Less than 100 mg/dL   Normal
100–125 mg/dL   Prediabetic
Greater than 126 mg/dL   Diabetic

(The reference ranges used for lab tests including optimal ranges are taken from Life Extension, Disease Prevention and Treatment)[37]

An optimal range of 70–85 mg/dL is recommended by the Life Extension researchers.[38]

Lipid Profile (standard)

The presence of fats in the blood is referred to as lipids. Fats are another source of fuel for the body and are also important components of cell membranes and certain hormones. Lipids are transported through the blood stream in the form of lipoproteins. This panel shows the levels of lipids present in the blood and should be interpreted as a screen for the risk of coronary heart disease, stroke, hardening of the arteries, and other metabolic issues. When results persist out of reference ranges set by the National Cholesterol Education Program (NCEP), further in-depth lipoprotein analysis should be done. This is because the functions involved with lipid metabolism that includes transport, utilization and the removal of lipids are complex, and several organs are involved[39]. A 12 hour fast is required for this test.

A standard lipid profile includes @ HDL cholesterol, LDL cholesterol, @ triglyceride, total cholesterol, and ratio total cholesterol/HDL cholesterol.

@HDL Cholesterol (High-density lipoprotein)

You may have heard of HDL as the "good" cholesterol. The HDL cholesterol is like a scavenger that removes oxidized cholesterol from your arterial walls and transports it directly to the liver. The liver manages the recycling or disposal of excess cholesterol.[40] Achieving an HDL number in the optimal range should be one of your goals.

Reference Range:
Normal   40–59 mg/dL
Optimal   Greater than 50 mg/dL

LDL Cholesterol (Low-density lipoprotein)

You may have heard of LDL as the "bad" cholesterol. Studies have shown that elevated levels of oxidized LDL cholesterol can infiltrate and damage the arterial walls, which can lead to heart disease.[41]

Reference Range:
0-99 mg/dL
Optimal   Less than 100 mg/dL

@Triglycerides

Triglycerides are lipoproteins synthesized by the liver and serve as a long-term source of energy storage. Measurements are used to decide the risk of developing heart disease, nephrosis and other disorders involving lipid metabolism.[42]

Reference Range:
Normal   0–149 mg/dL
Optimal   Less than 80 mg/dL

Total Cholesterol

Cholesterol is the major component of LDLs and a minority component of HDLs. Measurements are used to determine the risk of heart disease, diabetes, kidney and liver disease.[43]

Reference Range:
Normal   100–199 mg/dL
Optimal   160–180 mg/dL

Ratio Total Cholesterol/HDL Cholesterol

This calculation is used to determine the risk of coronary heart disease. Achieving an optimal level of HDL cholesterol (the "good" cholesterol) can decrease the possible risk for coronary heart disease when the ratio of total cholesterol to HDL cholesterol is calculated.[44]

Reference Range:

Men	Women	
3.4 mg/dL	3.3 mg/dL	½ Average Risk
5.0 mg/dL	4.4 mg/dL	Average Risk
9.6 mg/dL	7.1 mg/dL	2 Times Average Risk

Optimal

Men	Women
Less than 3.4 mg/dL	Less than 3.4 mg/dL

@Hemoglobin (Hgb) or Complete Blood Count (CBC)

Hemoglobin is the oxygen-carrying component of your red blood cells. This test is used to measure your hemoglobin level as might be reflected in your energy levels. It will reveal if you are anemic (low hemoglobin) or developing any other health issues.

Reference Range:
12.5–17.0 g/dL Men   11.5–15.0 g/dL Women

Optimal level the upper end of the reference range.

Oftentimes, instead of the hemoglobin test, your physician may order a Complete Blood Count (CBC). The CBC includes the hemoglobin and more. It is a group of tests that gives a snapshot of the blood's immune force: white blood cells, red blood cells, hemoglobin, and platelets. This test is used to detect disorders such as anemia, leukemia, and infections (viral or bacterial) and to assist in managing medications and chemotherapeutic decisions.[45]

@Vitamin D

Vitamin D has become one of the most talked about vitamins in the health industry. This is due to the extensive research revealing how essential this vitamin is to the body. Previously, it was believed that vitamin D was linked to gut and bone diseases. We now know that it is linked to almost every organ of the body, making this test one of the most reliable nutritional tools in wellness screens. When you don't have optimal levels of vitamin D, your body becomes vulnerable to developing diabetes, osteoarthritis, hypertension, cardiovascular disease, metabolic syndrome, depression, and cancers of the breast, prostate, and colon.[46]

Reference Range:
32–100 ng/mL
Optimal Level   50–80 ng/mL[47]

@ Glycated Hemoglobin (Hemoglobin A1C)

The hormone insulin (produced by the pancreas and triggered by carbohydrates in food) acts as a gatekeeper to allow the glucose into the cells without resistance. The glucose (sugar) released from foods binds to the hemoglobin in the blood as it is shuttled to areas of the body that require it. The hemoglobin is known then as glycated hemoglobin. When the body is working optimally, hemoglobin distributes this glucose throughout the body to be used as a source of energy.[48]

This test is helpful for accuracy based on previous increased fasting glucose levels, your age, or health history. It "looks back" two to three months at the levels of glycated hemoglobin and can indicate if the glucose distribution cycle has been disrupted.

Reference Range:
4.8%–5.6% Nondiabetic
Optimal Less than 4.5%
5.7%–6.4% Increased risk for Diabetes
Greater than 6.5% Diabetes
Less than 7.0% Glycemic control for adults with diabetes

Below are the remaining laboratory tests included in a Comprehensive Metabolic Panel (CMP). These equally important tests can reveal an all-inclusive glimpse of your overall health.

Liver function: AST (SGOT), ALT (SGPT), LDH, total bilirubin, alkaline phosphatase

Kidney function: BUN, BUN/creatinine ratio, creatinine, uric acid

Blood protein levels: total protein, globulin, albumin, albumin/globulin ratio

Blood mineral levels: calcium, sodium, potassium, phosphorus, iron, chloride

Fluid and pH (Acid–Alkaline) balance: Sodium, Potassium, Chloride, CO2 *These four electrolytes work together to influence general cardiac function (potassium, chloride), fluid balance (sodium), acid–alkaline balance, (CO2).*[49]

By now, you may have noticed that some of the tests listed above with the @symbol are markers directly associated with metabolic syndrome. Hence, the importance of knowing your numbers and implementing your preventive health plan. Here are the numbers associated with the *risk factors for metabolic syndrome.*[50]

- High Blood pressure: Avoid a blood pressure of 130 mm Hg/85mmHg or greater.
- Increased abdominal body fat: Avoid a waist circumference 40 inches or above if you are an adult male and 35 inches or above if you are an adult female.
- Elevated blood glucose: Avoid a fasting blood glucose of 100 mg/dL or greater.
- Lipid levels: Try to achieve an HDL cholesterol above 50mg/dL. Avoid triglyceride levels of 150 mg/dL or greater.

Depending on your health history and the initial results of lab tests done, your results may provide what is referred to as your baseline numbers. By continuously monitoring your health, you can work with your primary care doctor if any of your results fall out of the reference range. This can help to identify the cause, especially if there are accompanying health symptoms. So, it is important to have a comprehensive wellness screen done from the start. With your lab numbers and health history, additional tests or scans may be recommended for further guidance as precautionary measures.

Supplementary Lab Testing

So, you've completed your wellness lab tests, here are four examples that may occur:

1. All your lab results fall within or close to their normal reference ranges and you feel healthy overall.
2. All your lab results are normal; however, your BMI, blood pressure, or both are of concern.
3. Some of your lab results fall out of their normal reference ranges, and you don't feel 100 percent.
4. Some of your lab results fall out of reference range, but you feel healthy overall.

Although there are numerous tests that can be done to further probe into various health predicaments, with the guidance of your primary care doctor, any abnormal lab results may first be repeated depending on your medical history, general complaints, and for laboratory accuracy.

Here are a few of the accompanying lab tests that might be added when consistent out-of-range results are seen. A brief description follows each one. (Note that different situations may require different tests, as evaluated by your primary care doctor.)

Advanced Lipid Profile Test

This test is done when the LDL cholesterol (or HDL cholesterol) appears to persistently drift out of reference range even after changing diet, repletion with supplements, and modifying lifestyle habits (increasing exercise). This test will probe deeper to identify the lipoprotein particles making up the low-density lipids and the high-density lipids to provide a more detailed cardiovascular risk assessment.[51]

C-Reactive Protein (CRP)

This test can indicate underlying inflammation, infection, and stress within the body. This is an important marker to focus on when there is a chronic gum disease or cardiovascular issues.[52]

DHEAS (Dehydroepiandrosterone Sulfate)

DHEAS is the most common steroid hormone in the body produced mainly by the adrenal glands and used in the production of other hormones. Low levels of DHEAS have been linked to heart disease, abnormal cholesterol levels, depression, inflammation, immune disorders, schizophrenia, Alzheimer's disease, diabetes, and osteoporosis.[53]

Homocysteine

Homocysteine is another marker of inflammation and is linked to cardiovascular disease, stroke, Alzheimer's, hearing loss, and even migraine headaches. Homocysteine is an amino acid that results from the breakdown of animal protein during digestion. Vitamins B2, B6, and B12, when present in food, work together to help remove and reduce homocysteine through a metabolic chemical process. If homocysteine accumulates in high levels, it can inflict damage to the lining of the arterial walls and other cells of the body. Most individuals with high levels of homocysteine respond well to supplementation with vitamin B2, B6, and B12. There are, however, about 15–20 percent of the North American population that are resistant to this type of nutritional intervention because of an enzyme impairment within their metabolic system. This impairment can be identified with further lab testing, MTHFR genetic test. With the guidance of your primary care doctor, this problem can be corrected or controlled.[54]

Thyroid Stimulating Hormone (TSH)

Thyroid stimulating hormone (TSH) is associated with the thyroid function that directly affects your energy levels, metabolism, circulation, and brain function. Your primary care doctor may include this test with your screen if symptoms of weight management, abnormal mood swings, and unusual fatigue appear to be a lingering challenge.[55]

SpectraCell Micronutrient Test (MNT)

SpectraCell Micronutrient Test (MNT) is a specialized laboratory test that can determine if nutrient deficiencies are sabotaging your health and can help identify subclinical nutrient deficiencies that might be caused by factors beyond diet. Some of these factors might be teeth and gum health, metabolism, gut health, advancing age, disease conditions, and medications being consumed. Unlike most standard testing, MNT utilizes cells of the immune system, white blood cells, (T-cell lymphocytes) to evaluate the level of nutritional support present in your body. It reflects a period of four to six months in correlation to the average life span of a lymphocyte. This test is made up of seven components and in addition, offers an assessment of antioxidant deficiencies and the competence of your immune system.[56] Subsequently, you get a glimpse of the framework of your nutritional status. MNT is used by many integrative and conventional medicine physicians to assist with clinical evaluations, especially when patients have general symptoms common to chronic diseases such as fatigue and headaches.

Here are some of the micronutrients that are evaluated in this test and the body systems they support:[57]

Heart Health

Vitamin B6, vitamin B12, folic acid, vitamin E, CoQ10, calcium, magnesium, carnitine.

These micronutrients provide antioxidant defenses as they work together to support, energize and protect the heart.

Cardiovascular Support

Vitamin B3, vitamin B6, vitamin B12, and folic acid are all required for reducing homocysteine levels in the blood and protecting arteries and nerve fibers.

Bone Health

Vitamin D, vitamin B6, vitamin B12, folic acid, calcium, magnesium, and zinc assist in bone remodeling to ward off osteoporosis and other diseases that weaken the skeletal system.

Joint Support

Vitamin C, vitamin E, the fatty acid alpha-lipoic acid (ALA), and B vitamins all contribute to joint support and inflammation control.

Ocular Health

Vitamin C, vitamin E, vitamin A (including beta-carotene) are some of the micronutrients that protect and maintain good eyesight by preventing cataracts and macular degeneration.

Liver Health

Vitamin C, cysteine, N-acetyl cysteine, iodine, selenium, vitamin B2, and vitamin B3 enhance liver function and optimize levels of glutathione, which in turn helps cells fight off toxic challenges.

Metabolic Health

Vitamin B3, vitamin B6, vitamin B7, vitamin B12, vitamin E, coenzyme Q10, chromium, magnesium, and zinc all help the body handle your daily sugar intake, keeping systems responsive to insulin and restoring lost insulin sensitivity.

Two evaluations produced by the MNT results, Spectrox® and Immunidex, provide an in-depth view of your nutritional status. Spectrox® measures the ability of your cells to defend against and survive oxidative stress, (recall oxidative stress in chapter 1) and gives the antioxidant capacity of your lymphocytes. Immunidex gives an overall score of how well your immune system can respond not only to external threats such as allergens or pathogens, but also to internal threats such as tumors.

With this tool you and your primary care doctor can create a plan for repletion when necessary, through diet and targeted supplementation. This can avoid your system becoming vulnerable to health problems and long-term disease processes. Let's take a closer look at some of the foods that work with your body to repair, heal, and maintain a healthy status.

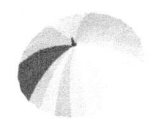

3

Nutrition Overview – Armor for Your Health

Can you recall what you've eaten over the past 24 hours? The Western diet and habits have been changing over time, but the nutritional needs and lifestyle for achieving optimal health have not changed. In this chapter, I share some of the basics of nutrition and the foods that supply it.

Achieving amazing health is the groundwork to a robust and accomplished life. What you eat, and drink will help to create the armor for your health which in turn will affect your overall lifestyle and the people around you.

Nutrition is directly linked to metabolism and sustained energy, which are the foundations to achieving a healthy weight, reducing food cravings, and maximizing your energy reserves. These three important aspects can be achieved by knowing the basics of nutrition. Using this knowledge will help you become responsible for your health and budget properly when purchasing the necessary foods to achieve a better lifestyle. Unintentionally, you will develop long-term healthy eating habits and not have to feel guilty when you deviate occasionally, which is normal.

Food supplies the body with the calories and nutrients for energy, growth, repair, and reproduction. We all share the same goals of wanting to keep our bodies fit to be able to make the greatest use of this gift of life. Yet, the seven key risk factors and behaviors that can lead to heart disease, stroke, and metabolic syndrome, if you recall from chapter 1, smoking, physical inactivity, low-nutrient diet, abnormal lipid levels, high blood pressure, diabetes and increased waist circumference, showed dismal statistics. What are the culprits to this multifaceted problem and how can you avoid becoming another statistic? There appears to be two common, underlying factors related to these risks: (1) the ***choices*** you make regarding what you eat and (2) your ***lifestyle habits*** (discussed more in Chapter 5).

Nutrition Overview

When you sit down to eat, is your meal normally a blend of foods in a variety of colors? Do the colors come from vegetables, grains, nuts, fruits, leafy greens, fish, poultry, and other meats? If so, these are considered whole foods (not produced in a factory) and are nutrient dense and most appropriate for the body. Our bodies are geared toward living, whole foods. This is the reason meals prepared from whole foods are best for our health and should be our first choice when available.[58,59] However, your geographic location influences the availability of whole foods and you may need to include processed foods (produced in a factory). When that is the case, you need to understand what the food labels reveal about the foods to make the best choices.

American Institute for Cancer Research (AICR) found that Americans are not getting the recommended 5 or more daily servings of fruits and vegetables needed to support a healthy status.[60] This might be related to our reliance on the processed food industry that has created a variety of foods, some more highly processed than others, that cannot replace the nutrient contents derived from whole foods. Do most of your meals come from processed foods and not from whole foods?

Whole Foods

Whole foods are vegetables, fruits, leafy greens, grains, fish, poultry, and other meats that come from farmed plants and animals. They are not produced in a factory.

Processed Foods

Processed foods, including processed snacks and beverages, are produced in a factory and are packaged with food labels. Some processed foods are so highly processed that they might have been once whole foods but have been transformed into entirely different products with artificial preservatives, colors, and flavors solely to capture our sense of taste. Once our taste buds are triggered we develop cravings to consume even more. These highly processed foods have very little nutrient content, water (except for beverages), or fiber. Trans fats (a type of unhealthy fat) have been incorporated into some of these foods to increase flavor and prolong shelf life. Most of these highly processed foods and sugary drinks will satisfy your immediate hunger and thirst but will not nourish your cells. The chemical makeup that provides information to your cells from these foods can adversely affect your health without creating immediate symptoms. You may have to eat highly processed foods several times before realizing that you are experiencing an adverse health reaction—you may even notice that you can no longer fit into your favorite jeans. Some examples of highly processed foods are preparations made from refined grains (white flour), refined sugar, processed meats, and refined cooking oils:

- Donuts
- Cookies
- Crackers
- Chips
- Macaroni and "cheese"
- Hot dogs
- Sausage mixtures
- Bacon
- Lunch meats
- Sodas, juice drinks, sweetened teas
- Imitation butter spreads, refined cooking oils, salad dressings

- Packaged sauces
- Sugary boxed cereals

The above-mentioned preparations are often referred to as *caloric-dense* foods. These highly processed foods may have increased caloric content with few nutrients. Thus, you should avoid highly processed foods whenever possible.[61]

Minimally processed foods, such as frozen meats (e.g., poultry, fish, beef, pork), fruits and vegetables, will contain most of the original nutrients and are referred to as *nutrient dense.* There are also canned foods that maintain some fiber and nutrient content but may have added salt and sugar. You can identify this information when you take the time to read labels attached to processed foods. Having said this, I have concluded from my personal research that not all processed foods are unhealthy. Many food manufacturers have made changes to reduce health-threatening ingredients in their food manufacturing process. However, you need to become familiar with the ingredients that can threaten your health and learn to identify the best choices when available. (See Helpful Websites). Let's take a close look at Nutrition Facts labels and how they can serve you.

The Nutrition Facts Label

The Nutrition Facts label can be your shopping guide to make the best choices. You can be easily misled by the appealing, colorful packaging which also applies to convenient and grocery store prepackaged meals. You may want to start by looking at the **ingredients** in the item you plan to purchase. This information is sometimes placed above the Nutrition Facts label, below it, on the side, or on the opposite side of the label. Depending on the food item, the shorter the list of ingredients, the better it is for you. If you find ingredients listed that you cannot pronounce, chances are they might be preservatives or artificial flavors you need to avoid. Your smartphone can help you identify unknown ingredients. Check for and avoid food items with ingredients such as high fructose corn syrup, chemical preservatives, artificial dyes and flavors, and foods with added sodium, sugar, and fat. The added sugar might be listed under the names of dextrose, sucrose, fructose, honey, or corn syrup. When selecting a boxed cereal, try to find one with less than eight grams of sugar per serving and with a recognizable, short list of ingredients.[62]

Note the type of fat present in the food item. If saturated fat is present (other than pure, unrefined coconut oil), the item should be eaten in moderation. Saturated fat from animals can raise your cholesterol and triglyceride levels when eaten regularly. Avoid foods that list trans fats (hydrogenated oils) on the label because trans fats are not good for the body.

Let's use this example taken from a box of frozen, uncooked, fish fillets to take a line-by-line look at the information provided on Nutrition Facts labels. This example is intended to help you become familiar with the layout of facts so that you can make informed decisions. If you have a processed food item on hand, you may want to compare that Nutrition Fact label with the example shown here, as you read along.

These images are for illustrative purposes of the Nutrition Facts Label. Despite modifications made to the Nutrition Facts Label by the Food and Drug administration to encourage consumers to make informed choices, one can only do so after understanding the concepts connected to nutrition and taking the time to read labels.

Nutrition Facts

Line 1 → Serving Size 5.2 oz. (146g/about 1 fillet)
Line 2 → Servings Per Container about 6

Line 3 → **Amount Per Serving**

Line 4 → **Calories** 140   Calories from Fat 30

Line 5 → **%Daily Value ***

Line 6 → **Total Fat** 3.5g   **5%**

Line 7 → Saturated Fat 1g   **5%**

Line 8 → Trans Fat 0g

Line 9 → **Cholesterol** 55mg   18%

Line 10 → **Sodium** 360mg   15%

Line 11 → **Total Carbohydrate** 2g   1%

Line 12 → Dietary Fiber 0g   0%

Line 13 → Sugars 0g

Line 14 → **Protein** 25g   50%

Line 15 → Vitamin A 2%   •   Vitamin C 4%
Line 16 → Calcium 2%   •   Iron 4%

*Percent Daily Values are based on a 2,000-calorie diet. Your daily values may be higher or lower depending on your calorie needs.

Line			2,000	2,500
Line 17		Calories	2,000	2,500
Line 18	Total Fat	Less than	65g	80g
Line 19	Saturated Fat	Less than	20g	25g
Line 20	Cholesterol	Less than	300mg	
Line 21	Sodium	Less than	2,400mg	
Line 22	Total Carbohydrate		300g	375g
Line 23	Dietary Fiber		25g	30g
Line 24	Protein		50g	65g

Line 1: The serving size for this package is one 5.2-ounce fillet. Compare this to Line 2 for the total number of servings in the package. One serving represents the numbers in Lines 4–16. If you plan to eat two or three servings at one time, multiply each of those numbers accordingly.

This line is also important when selecting beverages. ***Four grams (g) equal one teaspoon of sugar, which supplies approximately 16 calories.*** Some beverages (e.g., sodas and juices) come in 12-ounce containers containing two servings. Take note of the number of grams of sugar in one serving and do the math before consuming the entire item in one sitting. Beverages and boxed cereals are frequent sources of extra calories.

Nutrition Facts

▶ Serving Size 5.2 oz. (146g/about 1 fillet)
Servings Per Container about 6

Amount Per Serving

Calories 140   Calories from Fat 30

%Daily Value *

Total Fat 3.5g	**5%**
Saturated Fat 1g	**5%**
Trans Fat 0g	
Cholesterol 55mg	**18%**
Sodium 360mg	**15%**
Total Carbohydrate 2g	**1%**
Dietary Fiber 0g	**0%**
Sugars 0g	
Protein 25g	**50%**

Vitamin A 2%   •   Vitamin C 4%
Calcium 2%   •   Iron 4%

*Percent Daily Values are based on a 2,000-calorie diet. Your daily values may be higher or lower depending on your calorie needs.

	Calories	2,000	2,500
Total Fat	Less than	65g	80g
Saturated Fat	Less than	20g	25g
Cholesterol	Less than	300mg	
Sodium	Less than	2,400mg	
Total Carbohydrate		300g	375g
Dietary Fiber		25g	30g
Protein		50g	65g

Line 2: This package contains six servings.

Line 4: Each serving supplies 140 calories, 30 of which come from fat. If you are going to eat more than one serving, compare this information with Line 18 to assess your approximate intake of fat calories and then consider if additional food items can be added to balance this meal.

Nutrition Facts

Serving Size 5.2 oz. (146g/about 1 fillet)
Servings Per Container about 6

Amount Per Serving

Calories 140	Calories from Fat 30

	%**Daily Value** *
Total Fat 3.5g	5%
Saturated Fat 1g	5%
Trans Fat 0g	
Cholesterol 55mg	18%
Sodium 360mg	15%
Total Carbohydrate 2g	1%
Dietary Fiber 0g	0%
Sugars 0g	
Protein 25g	50%

Vitamin A 2%	•	Vitamin C 4%
Calcium 2%	•	Iron 4%

*Percent Daily Values are based on a 2,000-calorie diet. Your daily values may be higher or lower depending on your calorie needs.

	Calories	2,000	2,500
Total Fat	Less than	65g	80g
Saturated Fat	Less than	20g	25g
Cholesterol	Less than	300mg	
Sodium	Less than	2,400mg	
Total Carbohydrate		300g	375g
Dietary Fiber		25g	30g
Protein		50g	65g

Line 5: According to U.S. Department of Agriculture (USDA) Dietary Guidelines, the percent daily value of a nutrient/ingredient seen under this heading is related to a meal plan of 2,000 calories per day. *Twenty percent or above is considered high (which might be a "red flag" to avoid depending on the food item), and five percent or lower is considered low.*[63,][64] *You want your percentage of daily nutrients such as protein, vitamins, minerals, and fiber to be on the high end; saturated fat, sodium, and sugars on the low end.* According to USDA Dietary Guidelines,[65] this recommendation of 2,000 calories per day, pertain to individuals who are active, and of average size. If you tend to be less active, but of average size, you may want to consider consuming fewer calories daily to maintain a healthy weight. *This is where knowing which foods supply maximum nutrients with fewer calories can benefit you.*

Nutrition Facts

Serving Size 5.2 oz. (146g/about 1 fillet)
Servings Per Container about 6

Amount Per Serving

Calories 140	Calories from Fat 30
	%Daily Value *
Total Fat 3.5g	5%
Saturated Fat 1g	5%
Trans Fat 0g	
Cholesterol 55mg	18%
Sodium 360mg	15%
Total Carbohydrate 2g	1%
Dietary Fiber 0g	0%
Sugars 0g	
Protein 25g	50%

Vitamin A 2%	•	Vitamin C 4%
Calcium 2%	•	Iron 4%

*Percent Daily Values are based on a 2,000-calorie diet. Your daily values may be higher or lower depending on your calorie needs.

		Calories	2,000	2,500
Total Fat		Less than	65g	80g
Saturated Fat		Less than	20g	25g
Cholesterol		Less than	300mg	
Sodium		Less than	2,400mg	
Total Carbohydrate			300g	375g
Dietary Fiber			25g	30g
Protein			50g	65g

Line 6: The total fat content in one serving is 3.5 grams. When you compare 3.5 grams with the information given in Line 18 (65 grams allowed per day, when consuming 2,000 calories), it amounts to approximately 5 percent of the daily value of fat as given under the %Daily Value.

(Note the amounts shown on Lines 6–14, on the left side of the label with corresponding % daily values represent one serving). Percentage results are derived using the data given in Lines 18–24 in column 1 (based on a 2,000-calorie diet).

According to AICR's "Guide to the Nutrition Facts Label," the recommended daily intake of calories that come from fat should be approximately 30–35 percent.[66] This item can be a good addition to a balanced meal.

Nutrition Facts

Serving Size 5.2 oz. (146g/about 1 fillet)
Servings Per Container about 6

Amount Per Serving

Calories 140   Calories from Fat 30

%Daily Value *

Total Fat 3.5g	**5%**
Saturated Fat 1g	**5%**
Trans Fat 0g	
Cholesterol 55mg	**18%**
Sodium 360mg	**15%**
Total Carbohydrate 2g	**1%**
Dietary Fiber 0g	**0%**
Sugars 0g	
Protein 25g	**50%**

Vitamin A 2%	•	Vitamin C 4%
Calcium 2%	•	Iron 4%

*Percent Daily Values are based on a 2,000-calorie diet. Your daily values may be higher or lower depending on your calorie needs.

	Calories	2,000	2,500
Total Fat	Less than	65g	80g
Saturated Fat	Less than	20g	25g
Cholesterol	Less than	300mg	
Sodium	Less than	2,400mg	
Total Carbohydrate		300g	375g
Dietary Fiber		25g	30g
Protein		50g	65g

Line 7: Each serving has one gram of saturated fat. When compared with Line 19, it amounts to 5 percent of the daily value (when consuming 2,000 calories). Less than 20 percent is a good value for low saturated fat intake.

Line 8: Each serving has zero grams of trans fats, which is a good choice for a meal.

Nutrition Facts

Serving Size 5.2 oz. (146g/about 1 fillet)
Servings Per Container about 6

Amount Per Serving

Calories 140	Calories from Fat 30

	%Daily Value *
Total Fat 3.5g	5%
Saturated Fat 1g	5%
Trans Fat 0g	
Cholesterol 55mg	18%
Sodium 360mg	15%
Total Carbohydrate 2g	1%
Dietary Fiber 0g	0%
Sugars 0g	
Protein 25g	50%

Vitamin A 2%	•	Vitamin C 4%
Calcium 2%	•	Iron 4%

*Percent Daily Values are based on a 2,000-calorie diet. Your daily values may be higher or lower depending on your calorie needs.

		Calories	2,000	2,500
Total Fat		Less than	65g	80g
Saturated Fat		Less than	20g	25g
Cholesterol		Less than	300mg	
Sodium		Less than	2,400mg	
Total Carbohydrate			300g	375g
Dietary Fiber			25g	30g
Protein			50g	65g

Line 9: Each serving has 55 milligrams of cholesterol. When compared with Line 20, this provides 18 percent of your daily value of cholesterol.

Line 10: Each serving has 360 milligrams of sodium. When compared with Line 21, this provides 15 percent of your daily value of sodium. When checking labels, avoid products with 20 percent or higher amounts of sodium. The recommended limit on sodium has been lowered to 2,300 milligrams according to AICR, the Institute of Medicine, and USDA Dietary Guidelines.[67] *For blood pressure control, even less sodium intake is recommended.*

Nutrition Facts

Serving Size 5.2 oz. (146g/about 1 fillet)
Servings Per Container about 6

Amount Per Serving

Calories 140	Calories from Fat 30

	%Daily Value *
Total Fat 3.5g	5%
Saturated Fat 1g	5%
Trans Fat 0g	
Cholesterol 55mg	18%
Sodium 360mg	15%
Total Carbohydrate 2g	1%
Dietary Fiber 0g	0%
Sugars 0g	
Protein 25g	50%

Vitamin A 2%	•	Vitamin C 4%
Calcium 2%	•	Iron 4%

*Percent Daily Values are based on a 2,000-calorie diet. Your daily values may be higher or lower depending on your calorie needs.

	Calories	2,000	2,500
Total Fat	Less than	65g	80g
Saturated Fat	Less than	20g	25g
Cholesterol	Less than	300mg	
Sodium	Less than	2,400mg	
Total Carbohydrate		300g	375g
Dietary Fiber		25g	30g
Protein		50g	65g

Line 11: Each serving supplies two grams of carbohydrates, which can be compared with Line 22. Only a recommended goal is listed here. In this case, the recommended goal is 300 grams of carbohydrates if you are striving to remain on a 2,000-calorie daily intake. This food item allows additional small amounts of other carbohydrates to be added to balance the nutrient content (e.g., broccoli, green beans, brown rice).

Nutrition Facts

Serving Size 5.2 oz. (146g/about 1 fillet)
Servings Per Container about 6

Amount Per Serving

Calories 140	Calories from Fat 30
	%Daily Value *
Total Fat 3.5g	5%
Saturated Fat 1g	5%
Trans Fat 0g	
Cholesterol 55mg	18%
Sodium 360mg	15%
Total Carbohydrate 2g	1%
Dietary Fiber 0g	0%
Sugars 0g	
Protein 25g	50%

Vitamin A 2%	•	Vitamin C 4%
Calcium 2%	•	Iron 4%

*Percent Daily Values are based on a 2,000-calorie diet. Your daily values may be higher or lower depending on your calorie needs.

		Calories	2,000	2,500
Total Fat		Less than	65g	80g
Saturated Fat		Less than	20g	25g
Cholesterol		Less than	300mg	
Sodium		Less than	2,400mg	
Total Carbohydrate			300g	375g
Dietary Fiber			25g	30g
Protein			50g	65g

Line 12: This item offers no dietary fiber. The addition of vegetables, grains, and fruit can be added here to help achieve 25 to 30 grams of fiber as recommended by AICR.[68] Compare this information to Line 23.

Line 13: This item has no sugar. According to AICR, there is no recommended limit (or goal) for sugar consumption offered on Nutrition Facts labels.[69] There is room on this plate for a variety of small amounts of carbohydrates.

Nutrition Facts

Serving Size 5.2 oz. (146g/about 1 fillet)
Servings Per Container about 6

Amount Per Serving

Calories 140	Calories from Fat 30

	%Daily Value *
Total Fat 3.5g	5%
Saturated Fat 1g	5%
Trans Fat 0g	
Cholesterol 55mg	18%
Sodium 360mg	15%
Total Carbohydrate 2g	1%
Dietary Fiber 0g	0%
Sugars 0g	
Protein 25g	50%

Vitamin A 2%	•	Vitamin C 4%
Calcium 2%	•	Iron 4%

*Percent Daily Values are based on a 2,000-calorie diet. Your daily values may be higher or lower depending on your calorie needs.

	Calories	2,000	2,500
Total Fat	Less than	65g	80g
Saturated Fat	Less than	20g	25g
Cholesterol	Less than	300mg	
Sodium	Less than	2,400mg	
Total Carbohydrate		300g	375g
Dietary Fiber		25g	30g
Protein		50g	65g

Line 14: Each serving supplies 25 grams of protein, which is a good supply when compared with Line 24. If you are very active, such as a weightlifter, divide your weight (pounds) in half to determine your approximate amount of protein in grams. For example, if you weigh 140 pounds, your daily approximate goal of protein intake should be 70 grams.[70] A sedentary lifestyle requires less protein. Protein can be obtained from legumes, vegetables, nuts, meats, and dairy.

Nutrition Facts

Serving Size 5.2 oz. (146g/about 1 fillet)
Servings Per Container about 6

Amount Per Serving

Calories 140	Calories from Fat 30
	%Daily Value *
Total Fat 3.5g	5%
Saturated Fat 1g	5%
Trans Fat 0g	
Cholesterol 55mg	18%
Sodium 360mg	15%
Total Carbohydrate 2g	1%
Dietary Fiber 0g	0%
Sugars 0g	
▶ **Protein** 25g	50%

Vitamin A 2%	•	Vitamin C 4%
Calcium 2%	•	Iron 4%

*Percent Daily Values are based on a 2,000-calorie diet. Your daily values may be higher or lower depending on your calorie needs.

		Calories	2,000	2,500
Total Fat	Less than		65g	80g
Saturated Fat	Less than		20g	25g
Cholesterol	Less than		300mg	
Sodium	Less than		2,400mg	
Total Carbohydrate			300g	375g
Dietary Fiber			25g	30g
Protein			50g	65g

Lines 15 & 16: This is the percentages of vitamins and minerals found in each serving. According to AICR, "Manufacturers are required to list vitamins A and C and the minerals calcium, and iron" when present.[71] Other vitamins may be listed if a food is fortified with them. No claim is made about them unless the manufacturer chooses to do so.

This food example does not meet the daily percentages of these vitamins and minerals as recommended by the Food and Nutrition Board.[72] A reliable source of these vitamins and minerals can be added with fruits and vegetables, as well as a multivitamin supplement.

Nutrition Facts

Serving Size 5.2 oz. (146g/about 1 fillet)
Servings Per Container about 6

Amount Per Serving

Calories 140   Calories from Fat 30

%Daily Value *

Total Fat 3.5g	**5%**
Saturated Fat 1g	**5%**
Trans Fat 0g	
Cholesterol 55mg	**18%**
Sodium 360mg	**15%**
Total Carbohydrate 2g	**1%**
Dietary Fiber 0g	**0%**
Sugars 0g	
Protein 25g	**50%**

▶Vitamin A 2%   •   Vitamin C 4%
▶Calcium 2%   •   Iron 4%

*Percent Daily Values are based on a 2,000-calorie diet. Your daily values may be higher or lower depending on your calorie needs.

	Calories	2,000	2,500
Total Fat	Less than	65g	80g
Saturated Fat	Less than	20g	25g
Cholesterol	Less than	300mg	
Sodium	Less than	2,400mg	
Total Carbohydrate		300g	375g
Dietary Fiber		25g	30g
Protein		50g	65g

Overall, this food item is a good choice in planning a meal because it allows you to add other carbohydrates (macronutrients and micro-nutrients). This will help you to meet or balance your daily caloric and nutritional intake unique to your lifestyle. This serving of fish allows room on the plate for two servings of vegetables, one serving of grains, and later some fruit. Keep in mind, your daily three meals (or four to five smaller meals) and snacks should provide your unique number of calories which will be determined by your activity level.

As of May 2016, the Food and Drug Administration (FDA) has modified the Nutrition Facts label to emphasize important areas for consumers to be aware of, to make informed choices.[73] Some of these modifications include a bold and much larger type font for words such as serving size, calories, and the capacity of one serving. The %Daily Values footnote has been modified to state "The %Daily Value (DV) tells you how much a nutrient in a serving of food contributes to a daily diet. 2,000 calories a day is used for general nutrition advice."[74] These label improvements will be seen on processed foods as they come to market.

Selecting Whole Foods

All foods supply energy in the form of calories required to sustain your body systems. But when you select whole foods (foods not produced in a factory), they provide calories and more– ingredients known as **micronutrients, macronutrients,** and **fiber**. These are the foundations that make up a balanced diet needed by your body. Understanding their makeup, function, and how to use them to create delicious meals will benefit you. Micronutrients include vitamins, antioxidants, phytochemicals, and minerals. Macronutrients involve the greater part of the overall diet and are made up of carbohydrates, proteins, fats, and water. Fiber is the structural part of vegetables, leafy greens, and fruits. These three components are largely found in fresh, whole foods. They might appear in reduced amounts in minimally processed foods and are nonexistent in highly processed foods.

For every gram of carbohydrate or protein eaten, four calories of energy are obtained. For every gram of fat, nine calories are obtained. Some whole foods supply more nutrients and fiber with fewer calories than others. Those that supply more nutrients and fiber with fewer calories are referred to as nutrient dense. Those that supply more calories with less nutrients and fiber are referred to as caloric dense. Examples of nutrient-dense foods are berries, beans, lentils, and green leafy vegetables; these should be your first choice when available. Examples of caloric-dense foods are white rice, potatoes, and foods made from white flour.

Micronutrients

Micronutrients (vitamins, antioxidants, phytochemicals, minerals), are critical for all tissue structures, including bones, skin, and hair, and are important in all metabolic processes. In addition, minerals are needed to support the balance of your internal blood pH and body fluids and to maintain nerve function. If you recall from chapter 2, many body systems require micronutrients for optimal function, and requirements are unique to everyone. ***It is important to have them included in our daily meals.*** Below are descriptions of micronutrients, their functions and some of their food sources.

Micronutrients—Vitamins

The Latin root word ***vita*** means life.[75] Vitamins are essential to life and are involved in all metabolic processes. Almost all vitamins are found in whole foods and quality supplements. The body cannot make them, except for vitamin D (cholecalciferol) and vitamin B3 (niacin). Vitamins are classified as fat soluble and water soluble. The fat-soluble vitamins are A, D, E, and K. To absorb fat-soluble vitamins from foods, you need to have consumed some fat in your meals and the digestive and absorption function of your gut is normal.

Vitamins B and C are the water-soluble vitamins. Vitamin B was originally found to be a group of vitamins called B complex, consisting of more than one vitamin B. Each B vitamin differs chemically and is individually important to the body. The B vitamins are referred to as one group because they are often found together in the same foods; however, some are present in larger amounts than others. B complex consists of B1 (thiamine), B2 (riboflavin), B3 (niacin or nicotinic acid), B5 (pantothenic acid), B6 (pyridoxine), B7 (biotin) and in lesser amounts choline, inositol, and para-aminobenzoic acid, B9 (folate), and B12 (cyanocobalamin). ***Vitamin C provides antioxidant support and is essential for collagen production, which is needed for healthy skin.***[76]

Combining a variety of whole foods into your meal planning can make all the difference in supplying your body with micronutrients that work with each other to support your suit of armor. Here are examples of food sources that supply some of the vitamins discussed above. Keep in mind that most of these foods also supply varying amounts of ***antioxidants, phytochemicals, and minerals.***

Vitamin A

Milk, eggs, liver, fortified cereals, fruits, and green vegetables such as broccoli, brussels sprouts, cabbage, asparagus, and avocado.

Vitamin B (B Complex)

Whole grains and enriched cereals, brewer's yeast, nuts, seeds, legumes, sweet potatoes, green vegetables (e.g., broccoli, brussels sprouts, cabbage, asparagus, kale), soybeans, avocados, fruits, eggs, dairy, salmon, tuna, shrimp, meat, poultry, pork, and organ meats.

Vitamin C (Ascorbic Acid)

Oranges, grapefruit, peaches, papaya, mango, berries, and apples.

Vitamin D

Eggs, liver, fish oils, fortified milk and cereals.

Vitamin E (Tocopherol)

Green leafy vegetables, wheat germ, eggs, nuts, seeds, and legumes.

Vitamin K

Green leafy vegetables, butter, eggs, pork, liver, and cod liver oil.

Micronutrients—Antioxidants

Antioxidants (and phytochemicals) are used by the body to protect against oxidative stress. Some vitamins, such as Vitamin C, also function as antioxidants.[77] Antioxidants are responsible for stabilizing or deactivating free radicals in the body before they can accumulate in large amounts to have a negative effect on your cells. (Recall chapter 1) Have you noticed the browning effect (oxidation) seen on sliced apples or sliced avocados when left exposed to the oxygen in air? A drizzle of lime or lemon juice (filled with vitamin C) will deter this process.

Micronutrients—Phytochemicals

Phytochemicals are substances found only in plants (in addition to the vitamins and minerals), that provide remarkable health benefits. Research has shown that eating an abundance of plant foods as part of our meals can protect us from four of the leading causes of death in the United States: cancer, heart disease, diabetes, and high blood pressure.[78]

Examples of food sources filled with antioxidants and phytochemicals are tomato-based products, berries, oranges, mangos, papaya, broccoli, bokchoy, cabbage, kale, brussels sprouts, turnips, and asparagus. Asparagus is rich in the phytochemical glutathione (a protein that can bind to fat-soluble toxins for removal from the body) and is referred to as the "master phytochemical" by Jeff Primack, author of *Conquering Any Disease: The Ultimate High-Phytochemical Food-Healing System*.[79]

Micronutrients—Minerals

Minerals are unique because plants and animals do not produce them; they come from the earth and the ocean. Plants get minerals from water and soil; animals and humans must consume plants to obtain these minerals.[80] Minerals are critical for the proper composition of our body fluids, blood and bone formation, and maintenance of normal muscle and nerve function. Minerals in food do not contribute directly to energy needs but play a role in metabolic pathways. Many chemical reactions take place during metabolic processes that allow the nutrients to be transformed or synthesized into other vital chemicals needed by the body.

An adequate balance of minerals helps to maintain the body's acid and alkaline balance. Ori Hofmekler, author of *Metabolic Mystery Tour*, emphasized that the body's metabolism can become sluggish when there is an "over acidity" environment indicating a minute drop in pH. This minute drop can make the body vulnerable to infection and disease.[81] Foods that contribute to the acidity of the body come from consuming mainly animal foods, grains, and dairy products. Foods that contribute to the alkalinity of the body come from plants, hence the need to know how to combine different foods in your daily meals to create an acid-alkaline balance that is needed to support optimal health. Minerals are further divided into **macro minerals** and **trace minerals.**

Macro minerals needed by the body are sodium, calcium, chloride, potassium, magnesium, and phosphorus. Potassium, sodium, and chloride play vital roles as electrolytes, which regulate the body's electrical charge. Ori Hofmekler added, "Electrical charge is necessary for all cellular metabolic functions, but especially for the assimilation of nutrients and the elimination of toxins". [82]

If you are athletically inclined and have experienced muscle cramps with the excruciating pain that accompanies them, you might need more salt in your diet, an increase in calcium or magnesium, and or, an increase in hydration.[83]

An optimal potassium intake is associated with a lower risk of stroke, protection against loss of muscle mass, preservation of bone mineral density, and reduction in the formation of kidney stones.

Food sources rich in macro minerals include green leafy vegetables, bananas, lentils, nuts, dairy, and sardines.

Trace minerals needed by the body are iron, copper, fluoride, iodine, selenium, cobalt, manganese, sulfur, zinc, and chromium. ***Every cell in the body needs magnesium and iodine. Selenium primes the body for assimilating iodine. Selenium also functions as an antioxidant that works in conjunction with vitamin E. All cells have receptors for iodine. Iodine is essential for thyroid function and to support breast and prostate health.***[84]

Food sources of trace minerals include fruits and vegetables grown in mineral-rich soil, fish and sea vegetables, beef from grass-fed cows, soybean flour, seeds, and nuts.

Antioxidants, phytochemicals, vitamins, and minerals work together to protect your cells from tissue damage, disease, and aging. Research has shown that with a constant supply of micronutrients and exercise, we can deter the early signs of aging and prevent the development of degenerative conditions such as arthritis, diabetes, heart disease, and some forms of cancer.[85, 86]

Macronutrients

Macronutrients comprise the greater part of the overall diet and include carbohydrates, proteins, fats, and water. Macronutrients are required in moderately large amounts. When the body breaks down macronutrients, carbohydrates are turned into glucose; fats into fatty acids, ketones and glycerol; and proteins into peptides and amino acids. Although energy in the form of calories is supplied from these three categories of macronutrients, carbohydrates are the body's primary source of energy, followed by fats (ketones). The body's muscle mass, made up of protein is used for energy only when carbohydrates and fats are depleted. These categories of foods supply our cells with the building "mortar" and fuel to sustain a healthy life.

Macronutrient—Carbohydrates

As mentioned earlier, energy is sustained with carbohydrates, the body's primary source of energy, thus making it an important component of your nutrition. Nature has supplied us with two forms of carbohydrates: complex and simple. ***Complex carbohydrates*** are termed complex because they are packed with ***fiber, vitamins, minerals, and phytochemicals, and come directly from the land.*** Some complex carbohydrates have more of these ingredients than others and are considered ***"good carbohydrates"*** because they provide more fiber and nutrients and fewer ***calories*** per serving. They are referred to as ***nutrient dense.*** Examples of high-fiber, complex carbohydrates are broccoli, kale, green beans, asparagus, spinach, grains, and preparations made from whole grains. Servings from these foods can be added to your plate in larger portions.

Simple carbohydrates are those that provide less fiber and nutrients, depending on the source, with more calories per serving, and are often referred to as ***caloric dense.*** Examples include fructose (fruit sugar), lactose (milk sugar), manufactured table sugar, jams, syrups, refined flour, and foods prepared from refined flour. Manufactured foods with processed sugars can be considered ***"bad carbohydrates"*** when ***eaten regularly*** and served in ***larger portions.*** Some of the manufactured simple carbohydrates, if not carefully monitored, provide calories that can quickly add up. The sugar found in fruits and milk however, is usually combined with other nutrients and is good for you. If you recall, one teaspoon of sugar supplies approximately 16 calories; two chocolate chip cookies supply approximately 90 calories, and a typical 20-ounce soda supplies approximately 250 calories. Manufactured sugar is hidden in many highly processed foods. ***Meals with increased simple carbohydrates might be the culprit for causing mood swings, food cravings and, in many cases, the subtle, driving force behind metabolic syndrome.***[87]

Macronutrient—Proteins

As you age, you tend to lose muscle and strength. Men seem to lose muscle faster than women. Proteins provide the essential amino acids to build cells for all organs, preserve muscle, and play a vital role in several neurological functions. They are the building blocks of all enzymes. Proteins are found in plant foods such as peas, walnuts, lentils, broccoli, kale, quinoa, nuts and in animal foods such as beef, lamb, poultry, pork, seafood, eggs, milk, and milk products. When broken down, protein is made of many types of amino acids. The amino acid leucine plays a role in preventing muscle loss. Leucine is found in higher amounts in animal foods, milk and milk products, and to a lesser extent in plant foods. Here are some examples of foods and their protein content.[88]

Foods with protein	Grams
5 oz. roasted chicken	43
5 oz. cooked steak	35
5 oz. tuna	43
1 egg	6
1 cup milk	8
1 cup cooked broccoli	5
1 cup legumes (beans)	15
2 slices whole wheat bread	5
2 T. peanut butter	9
2 slices of cheese	14

If you recall from chapter 2, protein from animal foods, when undergoing the digestive process, produce an amino acid called homocysteine that can become a powerful and harmful oxidizing agent if not converted into a less harmful amino acid. The vitamins B2, B6, and B12, if present in your foods, work synergistically to effectively perform that conversion function. Studies have shown that an increased level of homocysteine in the blood is responsible for the initial damage to the inner walls of the arteries that subsequently leads to the initiation of atherosclerotic plaque formation. High concentrations of homocysteine in the blood is also linked to heart attack, stroke, and Alzheimer's disease.[89] Another reason to have your meals balanced with servings of green leafy vegetables and legumes to maintain a high level of the B vitamins needed to lower homocysteine levels if present.

Macronutrient—Fats

Much has been written on the topic of fats in foods and why you should avoid some of them, eat some sparingly, and eat some regularly because they are essential to your health. Fats are vital to your overall health and bodily functions. Besides being a source of energy and providing a layer of insulation under the skin, your body needs fats to build and protect cell membranes. Your body also needs fats to create hormones that regulate your blood pressure and reduce inflammation and pain. Fats are important for brain function and are directly involved in receptor formation and nerve transmissions. If you recall, fats are needed in the gut for the fat-soluble vitamins A, D, E, and K to be absorbed. It is well worth your time to understand how this macronutrient works to support your health and which ones to incorporate into your meals every day.[90]

There are three different kinds of fats you can find in foods: saturated, unsaturated, and trans fats. Their molecular structures differ, and this determines the outcome in your body and why some are considered "bad" fats and some "good" fats. Understanding these basics will help you make the right choices with your meal planning.

Fats are found in whole foods (from nature) as well as in processed foods (manufactured). Saturated and unsaturated fats are found mainly in whole foods. Trans fats are found mainly in processed foods, with some additions of saturated and unsaturated fats.

Saturated Fats

Saturated fats are found in meats, poultry, eggs, dairy, and some plant foods (e.g., coconut). Due to their molecular structure, saturated fats derived from animal foods ***require digestive processes to occur before they can be absorbed into the intestinal capillaries.*** Studies have shown that when this fat is eaten frequently and in large proportions, it tends to raise LDL cholesterol, which is considered the 'bad' cholesterol.[91] This leads to an increased risk for heart disease, stroke, cancer, and diabetes.

The saturated fat derived from coconut, (plant food) however, is one exception to this health risk because its molecular structure is different from the saturated fat found in animal foods, making it easily digestible. Coconut fat is one of the most healing foods provided by nature when consumed in its ***unrefined form.*** Coconut fat contains ***lauric and caprylic fatty acids,*** which research has shown to be ***highly antiviral, antifungal, and antibacterial.***[92] Mother's milk contains caprylic fatty acid, hence the reason why mother's milk is so vital for newborns. It helps to protect babies from infection while their immune systems are still developing.

Both animal fat and coconut fat are ***solid*** at room temperature. They can withstand high temperatures during cooking and do not break down chemically to have a negative effect on the body.[93] However, animal fat should be used sparingly in cooking for the reasons mentioned above. When selecting coconut fat (oil when liquified) for cooking, be sure the label reads ***"unrefined."***[94]

Unsaturated Fats

Depending on the molecular structure, unsaturated fats can be monounsaturated or polyunsaturated. They are ***liquid at room temperature*** and are made up of omega fatty acids: omega-3, omega-6, and omega-9. The Omega-3 and omega-6 are sometimes referred to as essential fatty acids because the body cannot produce them on its own; they must be obtained through your food.

Omega-3 (polyunsaturated) consists of three fatty acids: ALA (alpha-linolenic acid), EPA (eicosapentaenoic acid), and DHA (docosahexaenoic acid). **Omega-3 fatty acids are important for brain**

function, serve as building blocks for prostaglandins (hormones that regulate blood pressure, control inflammation and pain, support energy production including fat burning), and reduce platelet aggregation and LDL cholesterol, which in turn helps to reduce arthrosclerosis risk factors. These fatty acids are found in variable concentrations in some foods. ALA is found in high concentrations in *chia seed, walnuts, hemp, pumpkin seed, flax seed, and milk and beef from grass-fed cows. Dark green vegetables, wheat, and barley grass products are chlorophyll rich and a good source of ALA.*[95]

EPA and DHA are found *only in cold water fish, krill, and ocean microalgae.* The oils and foods rich in these fats (e.g., cod liver and krill oil) also supply vitamin E to the body.

Omega-6 fatty acid (polyunsaturated) includes several fatty acids but mainly linoleic acid (LA). Omega-6 is needed to trigger the body's inflammation response when you are injured or sick; it also promotes cell growth during and after physical activity. Omega-6 fats can be found naturally in *nuts, seeds, eggs, and pure, unrefined vegetable oils (e.g., soybean oil).*

Omega-9 fatty acid (monounsaturated) contains oleic acid, which has proven to help lower LDL cholesterol. It is abundant in pure, unrefined olive oil, most nuts, and in avocado.

Research has shown that omega-3s and omega-6s work together to provide the health benefits mentioned above but should be balanced so that there are *more omega-3s and less omega-6s present in meals.*[96] Why? Because *an excess* of omega-6s can disqualify the benefits of the omega-3s during metabolism, and omega-6s can encourage inflammation in the body that can increase the potential for body fat deposits, type 2 diabetes, arthritis, and heart disease. The bottom line is this: create a healthy balance by consuming *more high-quality omega-3 polyunsaturated fats and less omega-6 polyunsaturated fats.* When *purchasing an oil, look for one labeled "unrefined." Oils that are not labeled as unrefined will most likely be refined, although they are never labeled as such.* Use these unrefined oils in salads and for making spreads. Avoid cooking with them because they break down easily when exposed to high heat and are prone to oxidation, which can cause free radical damage in your body.[97]

Trans Fats

Small amounts of trans fats can occur naturally in foods such as milk and meat products. But an artificial form of trans fats is created through a process that adds hydrogen to liquid vegetable oils that makes them solid. These artificially produced trans fats have been introduced to the food industry to enhance flavor and extend shelf life. They do just that and more. Studies have shown *artificial trans fats to be a great threat to your health.*[98] *Artificial trans fats elevate LDL cholesterol ("bad" cholesterol), lower HDL cholesterol, ("good "cholesterol), and increase the risk of developing heart disease, stroke, and type 2 diabetes.* The Harvard School of Public Health noted that 228,000 heart attacks and 100,000 related deaths might be avoided in the United States each year by removing this form of artificial fat from our foods.[99] Some food examples where trans fats can be found are stick margarines and other spreads, fried foods including donuts, baked goods including cakes with almost solid frosting, cookies, pie crusts, crackers, and even frozen pizzas. Because of the known negative effects of trans fats, they are prohibited from being included in foods in certain geographical areas in the U.S.[100] It will benefit you to pay attention to labels to identify if trans fats might be present, so you can avoid these foods as much as possible.

Jeff Primack, author of *Conquering Any Disease: The Ultimate High-Phytochemical Food-Healing System,* claims that neither of the two primary categories of fats, saturated and unsaturated, are "healthy" or "unhealthy."[101] Instead, he advocates the blend of foods is what makes it healing or harmful to health.

The bottom line - avoid cooking with vegetable oils at high temperatures or try using unrefined coconut oil. *When eating out decrease your intake of foods cooked with vegetable oils. Increase as much as possible, those foods rich in omega-3s, such as cold-water fish, walnuts, flax seeds, and unrefined olive oil.*

Macronutrient—Water

Water makes up 65–75 percent of the human body and is second only to oxygen in the order of importance to sustain life. Did you know feelings of fatigue can be a warning sign of dehydration? Water is needed to flush out wastes and toxins from the body and to make up the fluids that transport the "electrical" minerals. When the body is not receiving enough water, toxins tend to stagnate, hindering digestive and elimination processes, which can bring on feelings of fatigue. How many cups of water, tea, milk, coffee, or juice do you enjoy each day? Our daily intake of water should be approximately six to eight glasses per day, or more, depending on lifestyle. *Water, therefore, increases energy, improves skin complexion, enhances your immune system, and can help to promote weight loss.*[102, 103]

Fiber

Fiber is the structural part of plants, vegetables, fruits, and legumes. Having fiber in your meals helps with the regular detoxifying of the body through removal of waste and toxins. It does this by promoting regular stool elimination, which prevents digested food from sitting in the gut any longer than it should. If losing weight is one of your goals, including larger portions of raw or slightly cooked foods rich in fiber should be a requirement. *Fiber-rich foods take longer to chew and help you to feel full faster. Plus, they tend to be low in calories and fat and provide a slow release of glucose as digestion takes place.* The higher the fiber content, the faster the movement of food through the intestinal tract, decreasing the time for fat absorption (assuming your meal includes some fat). Fiber is needed by your gut microbiome (a topic that deserves a book of its own).

Research has shown that fiber plays a role in reducing the risk of heart disease, diabetes, and colon cancer.[104] The recommended daily intake of fiber is 25–30 grams.[105] Is that close to your daily intake?

As you age, there is a bigger demand for nutrients to maintain the body's systems at an optimal level. There are many age-related changes and decline in bodily functions that might occur such as: loss of lean muscle mass, loss of collagen in the skin, decline in neurologic function and memory; gastrointestinal changes that may bring about problems with absorption and metabolism. Hence the need for more nutrient-rich foods and quality supplements. Research has shown that with a constant supply of micronutrients, macronutrients, adequate rest, and exercise, we can deter the early signs of aging and prevent the development of degenerative conditions such as arthritis, diabetes, heart disease, and some forms of cancer.[106]

4

Metabolism and Sustained Energy

Metabolism

Metabolism is the constant breakdown and conversion of food into molecular structures. These structures are transformed into biochemical compounds that are used to repair and create new cells within the body systems. It involves the process of elimination of waste and metabolic by-products. During your daily activities, the body generates and releases energy. While you rest, growth and repair take place. Metabolism is constant and ongoing. It is regulated by hormonal messengers and the brain to sustain your respiration, digestion, elimination, and movements of fluids throughout the body. The thyroid gland, (a small structure at the base of the neck and a member of the endocrine system) is linked to the regulation of your metabolism and energy levels.[107] If you recall in Chapter 2, the test TSH is associated with the function of this gland.

The molecular structure of the foods you eat consists of biochemical essentials that are interpreted by your cells for use within the body. Some of the molecular structures coming from certain foods are extremely helpful (e.g. antioxidants, phytochemicals) as discussed in chapter 3 – Selecting Whole Foods. Others can be damaging if not combined and balanced with other foods. If you recall in chapter 2, an amino acid called homocysteine that results from the breakdown of animal protein during digestion can build up over time and cause damage to your cells if not chemically neutralized and removed during the metabolic process. Caloric-dense foods and beverages supply energy immediately. Nutrient-dense foods and beverages release energy slowly and over a longer time. As food is metabolized with the combination of oxygen to make energy, carbon dioxide and water, a small amount of oxygen is transformed into a hazardous form known as reactive oxygen species or free radicals (previously discussed in chapter 1). Besides this origination of free radicals, other free radicals might have derived from toxins generated from pathological states, or from external sources (air pollutants, cigarette smoke, exposure to x-rays, medications, industrial chemicals, and pesticides). As metabolism occurs, the nutrients found in foods with the assistance of your immune system, work constantly to neutralize and eliminate existing free radicals. Yes, there can be a battle of good and bad molecular structures within you and you may not be aware of this until the critical numbers show up in your lab results.

Sustained Energy

Have you ever paid attention to your body's responses when you are hungry? Does your patience tend to be short? Are your thought processing and reactions slowed down? Do you feel nearly overwhelmed by nervousness? Have you also noticed that once you eat, you return to your normal, smiling, and contented self? How does this all happen so fast? As metabolism takes place, different messages in the form of hormones and electrical signals are sent throughout your body with the updated status from the derived energy. Glucose, derived from carbohydrates (e.g., grains, broccoli, kale, green beans, fruit juice), triggers the release of insulin, a hormone secreted by the pancreas (another member of the endocrine system). This insulin serves as the doorkeeper for allowing glucose into your cells to continue promoting metabolism. Insulin is primarily secreted in response to carbohydrates in your meals. If your meals include mainly processed, simple carbohydrate foods (e.g., donuts, cookies, candy, sugary cereals, juice drinks, white bread), there will be a constant demand for insulin to regulate the surge of glucose present. If your meals include mainly a blend of whole foods that are complex carbohydrates and proteins (e.g., vegetables, green leafy salads, unrefined grains, fruits) with nutrient-dense essential fats, the glucose from these foods will slowly be released (demand for less insulin) at a stable level to satisfy your hunger for a longer time.

When there are no big demands from activity to utilize glucose present in the blood (besides the body's metabolic use), excess glucose is converted into fat and stored in different areas of the body for later use. When the energy stored as fat is needed, it is converted once more into usable energy. If there is a constant demand for large amounts of insulin brought on by caloric-dense foods, this excessive use can cause the pancreas to become defective over time. Also, insulin can become less effective in its function, a condition known as insulin cellular resistance.[108] A defective pancreas or insulin cellular resistance can lead to a buildup of glucose in the bloodstream with serious metabolic effects creating type 2 diabetes.[109] If this accumulation is not discovered and corrected medically, the excess glucose in the bloodstream would begin to disrupt other organs including the heart, eyes, and kidneys. It may take several years of insulin resistance for you to develop full-blown diabetes and you may never know until that day when you are rushed to a hospital emergency room and your lab tests reveal critical, life-threatening numbers.

To avoid this scenario, assess what you currently include in your meals. If they are constantly filled with processed foods and aren't nutrient dense or don't include the good fats, you may want to question your daily energy requirements. If you haven't thought about your energy requirements, you can estimate what that might be by reviewing the example given in the information in chapter 3, Nutrition Facts label. To maintain a healthy weight, would you qualify for a Daily Value (DV) of 2,000 calories coming from all your meals, snacks, and beverages? Or, a Daily Value of 2,500 calories? If you have concluded that you are not very active and of a smaller size, you may qualify for a daily value of 1,500 calories.[110] You can get an even more accurate estimate of your daily caloric requirements by visiting one of the many health websites that use a mathematical formula based on your age, activity level, and gender to calculate this number.

You may have the access capabilities to download health apps onto your smartphone. One that might be capable to monitor your daily activities and provide the approximate number of calories you burn during a 24-hour period. This knowledge will allow you to experiment with the foods that will be nutrient dense to feed your cells and at the same time support a healthy weight. Another health app available is one that offers exercise routines that you can use at home or while at work to boost your activity level. Many of these apps are free of charge, but others may require a small fee. Healthy weight ranges for men and women of various ages can also be found online, but always consider your waist measurements when viewing these healthy weight ranges. Another beneficial access to health websites is the variety of healthy recipes that can be retrieved in response to your tastes.[111] If you do not have access to the internet, a visit to your local library with this request should get you many of these answers.

Gary Taubes, author of *Good Calories, Bad Calories,* conveyed George Cahill's theory of fat accumulation in his lecture when he said, "Carbohydrate is driving insulin, is driving fat."[112] With the correct choices of food to accommodate your lifestyle, whether it includes a high level of activity or a low level of activity, your body can stimulate fat deposits to shrink accordingly. If you are unable to include moderate to vigorous activity in your daily lifestyle, then your diet requires scrutiny to align with your energy output. Your energy demands directly affect the fat storage you carry within. When this concept of sustained energy is grasped, you will begin to align your food choices with your lifestyle and you will no longer need to focus on counting calories.

As you age, there is a bigger demand for micronutrients to support metabolism and sustain energy. If you recall earlier (chapter 3, Mircronutrients), the requirements for micronutrients vary and are unique to everyone. It can be difficult to obtain optimal levels of micronutrients when relying on consuming whole foods. Hence, the addition of quality supplements in your daily regimen should be considered.[113]

Why Supplements Can Help

Have you wondered how much of various whole foods are needed daily to support a healthy body? As mentioned in chapter 1, your unique genetic and biochemical makeup together with your environment directly influence your health. Even though there is no replacement for a healthy, well-balanced diet, to achieve optimal levels of nutrients, the addition of superior, quality supplements can help to ensure you get the amounts needed for the "integration of immune system functions"[114] This will help also to avoid food cravings.

According to Dr. Ron Kennedy, author of Short History of Vitamins,[115] in the 1930s, scientific discovery confirmed the biochemical functions of vitamins and minerals and introduced the body's requirements for them. Since then, supplements have been commercially produced to enhance our daily, dietary intake of nutrients. In 1994, the Dietary Supplement Health and Education Act (DSHEA), was put into effect by U.S. Food and Drug Administration (FDA) to regulate the marketing of supplements.[116] The manufacturers and distributers are held responsible for ensuring that a dietary supplement is safe before it is marketed, and the FDA is responsible for acting "against any unsafe dietary supplement product after it reaches the market."[117, 118] In 2002, the American Medical Association encouraged all adults to supplement their diet with a daily multivitamin. This was based on the scientific evidence of their importance presented by Drs. Robert Fletcher and Kathleen Fairfield, a couple of Harvard researchers.[119]

Many manufactured supplements can be found on the market, but how can you tell which supplements are of good quality and provide the nutrient amounts stated on the label? There are independent testing companies that work to help the public identify the best quality, health and nutrition products on the market. One of them is Consumer Lab (CL). A label that bears the "CL" approval means the product has passed

CL's quality tests for properties that relate to potency, good manufacturing practices and looking for the presence of harmful levels of contaminants.[120] Another independent testing company is NutriSearch Corporation. This company specializes in the evaluation of supplement products in the global marketplace. A publication with current research and results titled, *NutriSearch Comparative Guide to Nutritional Supplements* is available to the public.[121] Their research incorporates stringent product analysis when evaluating supplement products. They check for label claims, adhering to the guidelines for good manufacturing practices, product efficacy, and they too look for the presence of harmful levels of contaminants. A rating standard from one to five (five the highest) is allotted to products that have met the NutriSearch level of scrutiny. Other resources for information on supplements are the Alliance for Natural Health USA and *The Physicians' Desk Reference for Nonprescription Drugs, Dietary Supplements and Herbs*.

The term Recommended Dietary Allowances (RDAs), as seen on supplement labels, refers to the recommended daily amount needed to protect from deficiency. The RDAs are developed by the Food and Nutrition Board at the Institute of Medicine of the National Academies.[122] There are many different RDAs for each nutrient because they vary by age, gender, and various conditions (e.g., pregnancy). Your goal is not only to prevent deficiency disorders but to maintain **optimal health**. Therefore, it is well worth your time and diligence to research the producer of the supplements you intend to purchase and not simply buy what is being marketed.

Another challenge you might face is determining whether your well-balanced diet is providing the expected amounts of important minerals. Lyle MacWilliam, author of *NutriSearch Comparative Guide to Nutritional Supplements*, noted, "Plants can't make minerals, they must absorb them from the soil—and without minerals, vitamins don't work." He added, "If important minerals are depleted from our soils, they are also depleted from our bodies."[123] To learn more about adequate levels of vitamins and minerals needed to sustain optimal health, see the Helpful Websites at the end of this book.

Vitamin D has been in the spotlight for its many roles in strengthening and supporting the immune system, heart, and liver, as well as metabolic health. Previously, the RDA for vitamin D was 400 international units (IU) per day; however, that has been increased to 1,000 IU per day and in certain cases up to 4,000 IU per day.[124] If you recall from chapter 2, Vitamin D level is now included in wellness screens and if found to be below the reference range, repletion is highly recommended.

The trace mineral iodine has its biological impact not only on the thyroid gland but also on several other tissues including the mammary glands, prostate gland, eyes, gut, arterial walls, cervix, and salivary glands. The RDA for iodine has also been increased from 150 micrograms (mcg) per day to 1,000 mcg per day.[125]

5

Another Type of Nourishment

What if there is an additional form of nourishment that energizes the body and mind but is not traditionally looked upon as nourishment? Could that be another piece to your health puzzle?

According to the Institute for Integrative Nutrition®, the term "primary food" is used to describe that additional form of nourishment that energizes the body and mind and nurtures your emotional well-being.[126] This nourishment is embodied by the resulting six aspects of your life:

1. A spiritual practice
2. Social interactions and strong relationships
3. Home cooking, health, and home environment
4. Career, finances, creativity, education
5. Regular physical activity
6. Joy

These categories integrate as you journey through life and, when balanced, are fulfilling and provide the "primary food" that feeds you—making the food you eat on your plate secondary, but essential. You don't know what the future has in store for you and whether your expectations for achieving certain goals in life will be met. How you react and continue with life in the event of positive or negative outcomes is what determines your ability to pursue a balance of "primary foods" to enrich your life.
When you wake up feeling refreshed and energized, you seldom

contemplate your biological existence. However, when you don't have the vigor to do your daily tasks or you are unable to mentally move beyond your stress and challenges, you are forced to focus on your psychological and emotional well-being. Your psychological, emotional, and social well-being are interwoven with your thoughts and actions. It is in your best interest to be aware of some uplifting practices and habits that can serve as the groundwork to protect and nourish your emotional and physical well-being.

Managing Puzzle Pieces

Let's start with an exercise called the "Circle of Life," taken from the Institute for Integrative Nutrition® (IIN®) that incorporates aspects of life that nourish your mind and body.[127]

1. Start by drawing a circle with a diameter of four to five inches.
2. Divide the circle into 12 sections. (See example on opposite page.)
3. Label the sections *Spirituality, Education, Creativity, Career, Finances, Health, Physical Activity, Home Cooking, Home Environment, Relationships, Social Life,* and *Joy.*
4. Place a dot on the line for each section to designate how satisfied you are with that part of your life. A dot placed on the line toward the center of the circle indicates dissatisfaction, while a dot placed toward the periphery indicates ultimate happiness.
5. After placing a dot on each line, connect the dots to view your circle of life.

"CIRCLE OF LIFE" EXERCISE ®

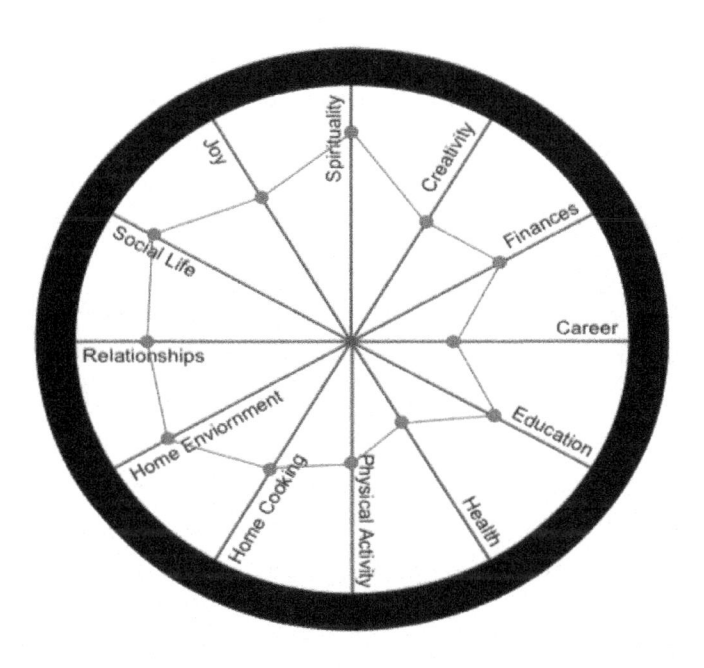

©2005 Integrative Nutrition Inc. (Used with permission.)[128]

You might already be aware of areas in your life in which primary food is absent or deficient and needs support, but now you have a visual guide of how it fits into your health puzzle. Your world and life are constantly evolving, and there might be times when many of these areas appear to be in disarray—this is normal. Even when you fail with endeavors, it is okay because you can turn things around with support and guidance. If your circle is not to your liking after completing the exercise for the first time, save the image and begin a plan to make your circle the way you would like it to be. Set a goal and then work out the details on paper for how you want to achieve it. Ask yourself why it is important to make a change and write down your answer. Then, plan your first step towards this change until it is accomplished. Write out the possible obstacles you may face and ways to overcome them. Share your goals and ideas with a few people in your life who will support you and keep you accountable.

Go forward with an action that you can accomplish in the first 24 hours. Then, set up your actions for the next seven days. Visualize what it will be like to succeed with your plan at hand. Work slowly to get results and to form habits with new behaviors. Return to this exercise in three to four months to note the changes. The improvements made will be felt even before visually seeing the change on your circle. Reward yourself in a mindful way for your achievements.

Working with these 12 aspects of the circle of life model will help to keep you motivated to take responsibility for your health. The following are a few suggestions of actions and habits to improve or help to develop a positive attitude, that is essential to managing stress and overcoming challenges. I hope this synopsis will spark your interest to dig further for answers that may be applicable to *your* life so that you can make adjustments where necessary or seek the required help to safeguard and nourish your emotional well-being.

Spirituality

Do you feel connected to an intangible force in this world? Research has shown that those who incorporate a spiritual discipline as part of their lifestyle and feel connected to a higher entity, such as Mother Nature, tend to show "qualities of love, honesty, patience, tolerance, compassion, a sense of detachment, faith and hope."[129] It is their belief that they have a purpose in this world, which in turn helps to create the emotional determination to carry on and seek solutions to challenging situations at hand.

Research has shown that a habit of quieting your thoughts each day, even if for just five minutes, can create a healing state for the body.[130] It is so easy to become wound up in a world of family, career, finances, and relationships that you can miss experiencing the "now." If this is not one of your habits, you may now want to include a quiet period in your daily schedule. Start with five minutes, then increase the time accordingly. Simply listening to calming music or connecting to nature around you might be one of your choices. First, select a time during the day that works best for you. It might be at the start or end of your day. Carve that time out for you. Try to observe your surroundings and avoid the chatter of your brain. Indulge in meditation, turning inwards to become aware of your breathing pattern as you bask within your being. Life is fragile and sacred. You may want to begin or end this calming period with gratitude. Count your blessings and be thankful for waking up to experience a new day with the gifts of your senses and having a place to live with meals and clean clothes. We tend to take these basics for granted until they are taken away through life's circumstances or events. How often do you show and express your gratitude to whoever might be supporting you in this area?

Social Life and Relationships

Do you offer support to others and tend to create relationships with those you can trust? As humans, we have an innate social desire to be happy and are nourished by communicating and interacting with our peers, building quality friendships, and experiencing mindful relationships. When we are shown appreciation either for helping others, contributing to our community, or providing financially for our family, we are fed with a reflective fulfillment. Do your relationships with your spouse, family members, or friends positively "feed" you, or do these relationships have adverse effects on your energy? This might be part of your evolving world and it is up to you to seek changes as needed. It's also okay to say "no" to others and tasks that can create stress that impede the balance of your circle of life.[131]

Home Cooking, Health, and the Home Environment

Putting together a plan for your nutritional and emotional well-being can be the best shield to protect you during life's journey and the challenge of maintaining optimal numbers. Despite having a sound nutritional plan, if you live in conditions where you don't feel safe (e.g., your life is threatened by a family member, coworker, neighbor, or someone you once trusted) your health will be affected. The fight-or-flight stress hormones produced by your body are needed during life-threatening situations. However, if circumstances in your life constantly trigger these stress hormones, and you are unable to control and balance these areas of your life, it might be time to speak up and seek help. Some situations may require professional help. Journaling (if this is not already one of your habits) will help you monitor what occurs at home and at work. Writing your thoughts on paper in response to various situations can help you adjust or pinpoint where improvements might be needed. You may have health issues related to the air you breathe, the water you drink, or the food you eat. Food and environmental allergies can also be discovered through journaling as you document changes that are occurring. In the case of possible food allergies, writing down everything you eat for 7 to 14 days and what reactions or symptoms you experience, might be able to correlate specific foods with changes in your mental and physical state. It is well worth your time to seek guidance from a professional if you need to make corrections for the sake of your health.[132]

Because life is unpredictable, you can never be totally prepared for all situations. However, in almost everything you do, preparation can alleviate fear and help you deal with some of the unexpected events in and around your home and community. Prepare a list of phone numbers to utilities such as gas, telephone, water, and garbage, the local police department, your primary care doctor, and the closest pharmacy and hospital. Also, make a list of phone numbers of those in your circle of family and friends whom you can count on for emotional support and guidance. Have this list readily available for emergencies. Work with your family to develop a strategy for dealing with stress and unexpected occurrences. Start your plan of preparedness by creating a list of items that are most important to take with you if you must evacuate your home.

Career, Finances, Creativity, and Education

Your emotional well-being is nourished when you are involved in a career that contributes to society with positive outcomes. When a job or service is well done regardless of the service rendered and respect is shown to others in your daily environment, the whole institution benefits.

Do you appreciate and are you passionate about the job you do? It is essential to your health to have a career that you enjoy and to be able to converse with and connect socially with your coworkers because this is where you spend most of your day.

Is the environment favorable to your health? If you suspect that your job is a risk to your health, but the paycheck keeps you from quitting, then you may want to speak with a career counselor to get ideas on how to assess your situation to bring about changes, if necessary. On the flip side of this, financial challenges can take a toll on your overall wellness. Maintaining a healthy level of stress about finances can safeguard not only your physical and emotional health but can also safeguard your relationships with those close to you. Learning how to manage your debt-to-income ratio, even on a modest income level will allow you to create a state of financial wellness. Studies have shown that money is an important asset to acquire, but its use for economic purposes has its limitations as the poet Arne Garborg so well stated:[133] "You can buy food, but not appetite; medicine, but not health; knowledge, but not wisdom; glitter, but not beauty; fun, but not joy; acquaintances, but not friends; servants, but not faithfulness; leisure, but not peace." Learning to have a balanced outlook on money and its purpose as a means to an end rather than an end itself can help to create an outlook of contentment amidst financial chaos.

The loss of a job could create recurring financial issues. Know that when this occurs, you are not alone; many find themselves on this path. There are solutions to these dilemmas. Don't feel that you should handle these issues without help from others. You might be surprised to learn your village hall, county office, or your community church can be a great resource to guide you to financial counseling and other support in this area. It might be necessary to start over (there is no shame in having to start over) with a new financial plan and regimen to avoid spending more than you earn.

Today in the United States, there are flexible companies willing to train new employees on the job. There are opportunities to develop new skills or build on what you already know by engaging in trade or professional programs offered by occupational institutions. Even an entrepreneurial pursuit might be possible with available guidance and finances to use your expertise and skills to help others. Many valuable lessons can be learned during these times, one of them is that you do not have to impress others to make them like you. Your outlook on life and determination to act and move on will help to bring about positive changes.

Physical Activity

Exercise is a crucial component in your circle of life and health maintenance. If your daily lifestyle does not include moderate activities, do you set aside time for planned exercise? If you tend to sit most of your day and exercise is foreign to you, here is what you might be missing: Exercise not only benefits the metabolic, cardiovascular, bone, and muscular system, it is also critical for promoting the creation of new brain cells to help reduce the risk of cognitive decline as you age. Exercise triggers the production of more endorphins in the brain and induces longer and more restful sleep that is needed to rebuild cells throughout the body. According to AICR, exercise "reduces infections—moderate workouts temporarily rev-up the immune system by increasing the aggressiveness of immune cells which may explain why people who exercise and eat a mixture of whole foods, tend to catch fewer colds." [134, 135]

AICR recommends getting at least 30 minutes of moderate physical activity daily and added that this activity can be broken into "10 or 15-minute segments for a daily total of 30 minutes to make it easier."[136] Some moderate activities may include brisk walking, jogging, swimming, cycling, wood chopping, weeding the garden, mowing the lawn, dancing to your favorite music, mopping floors, vacuuming, and working out at a gym. Vigorous activities may include basketball, racquetball, football, stair climbing, running, rowing, and almost all competitive sports.

If moderate physical activity or exercise is not part of your lifestyle, then select one or more of the activities suggested above and ***start*** a new habit. You may even want to add walking upstairs instead of taking an elevator or parking your car a mile away from your job. Set a goal to walk a mile or two each day and monitor how long it takes to do so. Plan to decrease that time by increasing your walking speed. Once you have accomplished that, set a new goal to increase the distance. As you improve, aim for 60 minutes of moderate activity or 30 minutes of vigorous activity at least three times a week.

An exercise program such as yoga is excellent for strengthening, toning, and stretching muscles. There are several forms of yoga that can be fast paced and intense or gentle and relaxing with meditation.

To achieve and maintain a weight that encourages long-term fat loss, Jonathan Bailor, author of *The Calorie Myth,* advises to "exercise in a way that activates your hormones."[137] Exercise resistance is the way to go rather than the number of times you exercise and the duration. He recommends a high-intensity interval training program that includes "eccentric" weightlifting moves, which are moves that "engage the hormone-shifting muscle fibers that help to regulate whole-body metabolism."[138] He explains that the muscle-extending moves will enable us to "generate more force and activate more of our fat-burning muscle fibers."[139] Bailor suggests leg presses, chest presses, seated rows, and overhead shoulder presses to accomplish this fat burning process.[140] You can add this form of exercise to your other aerobic activities because it requires no more than 10 minutes each time, twice a week. Research has also shown that this type of strength-training exercise helps to enhance memory and cognitive decline in aging adults even more so than aerobic exercises.[141] Therefore, combining an aerobic and strength training regimen, which may include yoga, can be an ongoing goal to achieve.

Joy

Do you deliberately schedule "joy" time into your weekly routine? Research has shown that it is important to fit fun or joy into your life.[142] This will create relaxation and help to replenish your emotional energy and state of calmness. By now you might have noticed that the above mentioned six aspects of your life contribute to the joy in your life.

Spending quality time with family and friends that may include activities such as dancing, fishing, relaxing at an ocean or lake, picnicking, watching a movie, experimenting with a new recipe, getting a massage, attending a performance or lecture, and many other outings can create another form of stress reduction for your mind and body.

If you would like to begin inexpensive, fun activities, your local library can be a resource to introduce you to local community events. An unexpectedly fun activity can be getting to know your city and state. First, make a list of the interesting places close by and those more than 25 miles away. Take the time to visit them as part of your family outings. Also, research has shown that laughter relaxes the blood vessels which in turn helps to improve blood circulation.[143] So, seek out humorous movies to enjoy either at home or at the theater.

6

Creating Your Unique Plate

What entices you to eat certain foods? Is it how they look, smell, or taste? Do you eat them because you know that they are healthy for you? Maybe it's a combination of all these things in addition to the knowledge that you prepared these foods yourself. Preparing and cooking your meals will give you control over what you consume. When planning your unique plate, you need to know how to blend whole foods (those not produced in a factory) and vary your portion sizes to create the energy and necessary pH balance for your body. You can also apply this practice when eating out. In this chapter, you will learn how to balance certain food groups to create your unique "plate" as suggested by American Institute for Cancer Research (AICR) and the method of Food Combining, as proposed at the Institute of Integrative Nutrition®.[144,145] I include examples of portion sizes to show how they influence your caloric intake. I reveal some of my practices for planning and creating nutritious, delicious meals, as well as on-the-run snacks and lunches. Your goal is to have these meals and snacks readily available to allow you to maximize nutrients and minimize calories during busy days. You may be surprised to learn how quickly calories can add up depending on the type of food consumed.

If you recall from chapter 3, the body needs "Carbohydrates" for energy to sustain an efficient metabolism based on activity, gender, and age; proteins to build and sustain muscle (not just the visually attractive biceps and glutes, but also the muscles of all the internal organs); vitamins and minerals to support muscle-building, and to resist/deter the aging process and water to flush out toxins and sustain biochemical processes. Where should you begin?

Knowing your approximate daily caloric requirement is beneficial in the beginning to understand how to create your unique plate. However, it is not required. As you develop a habit of eating whole foods, including more plant-based foods in your meals and snacks, counting calories will become a memory. The recommended 5 or more daily servings of fruits and vegetables by AICR is a good place to start.[146] Besides the nutritional benefits mentioned in chapter 3, **plant foods provide the most alkalizing components needed to help stabilize your internal acid–alkaline balance.** The acidity or alkalinity properties connected to foods are measured by the residue that is left in your body once the food is metabolized. For example, a lemon tastes sour or acidic, but once metabolized it leaves an alkaline residue. The foods that outwardly appear to be acidic foods are truly metabolically alkaline in the body. Foods such as grains, meats, and refined sugar are metabolically *acidic*. The ideal pH of your blood for optimal health is around 7.35, which is neither too acidic nor too alkaline but neutral. Research has proven that an acidic environment is more favorable to illness and disease; therefore, *your internal pH balance directly influences your state of health.*[147]

Whole foods, organic or conventionally grown, are available to most Americans amidst much debate. Why is this? Not too long ago, all foods were *organically* grown, that is, without the use of chemical-based fertilizers. The land was fertilized with manure and compost, and crops were rotated to allow the soil to regain its nutrients between cycles. Animals could graze on that land as part of the process without being fed antibiotics and growth hormones. This method added to the ecosystem that is vital to plants and the degree of nutrients found in them. Nowadays, conventional, non-organic farming may provide bigger crops, larger harvests (in less time) with reduced labor costs and more financial gain for those farmers. However, the synthetic, chemical-based fertilizers, industrial pesticides and artificial growth hormones utilized, are a threat to your health, even after meticulous washing. Continually eating meat, dairy products, poultry, eggs, from non-organic or conventionally farmed animals and crops, has been shown to cause cancer and other diseases.[148, 149] Many farmers have been returning to the organic way of farming because the demand has risen for food derived from grass-fed, cage-free animals raised without added hormones. Plus, consumers are willing to pay more for plant foods that are chemical-free. Shopping at some of the locally grown, organic farm markets might cost less than at some of the well-known Whole Foods markets. Moreover, the produce would not have traveled halfway around the world to get here. Currently, some of the popular chain stores in the United States (depending on your geographic location), such as Walmart, Target, and Aldi, carry both organic and conventionally grown whole foods, and their prices are very competitive. It is well worth your time to investigate whether these stores, or similar ones, are in your community.

"Clean" vs "Dirty" Foods

The Environmental Working Group has identified which fruits and vegetables derived from conventional farming contain the most residue chemicals and which ones are the least contaminated.[150, 151] Those with the most residue is called "dirty" because residues persist despite all the washing to remove the chemicals sprayed on these items. Those with the least residue is considered "clean" or may have very little residue after washing. It will take some initial diligence on your end to select the organic and conventionally grown foods you want to include on your food list to fit your budget. The term "eating clean" is sometimes used to describe consuming organically cultivated whole foods.

Here are the foods considered "dirty" and the foods considered "clean" referred to as "Dirty Dozen Plus" and "Clean Fifteen".[152]

The "Dirty Dozen Plus"

The "Dirty Dozen" plus are: Apples, celery, cherry tomatoes, cucumbers, grapes, hot peppers, imported nectarines, peaches, potatoes, spinach, strawberries, sweet bell peppers, kale/collard greens, summer squash.

The "Clean Fifteen"

The "Clean Fifteen" plus are: Asparagus, avocados, cantaloupe, sweet corn, eggplant, grapefruit, kiwi, mangoes, onions, mushrooms, papaya, pineapple, sweet peas (frozen), sweet potatoes, cauliflower

When shopping for organic food, not only do you want to see the label "Certified Organic" but also a produce code known as a PLU (price look up) code that confirms you are getting an organic product. Here is a list of PLUs you should become familiar with:[153]

4 Digit Code	5 Digit Code	5 Digit Code
Starting with number 3 or 4	Starting with number 9	Starting with number 8
Conventionally Grown	Organically Grown	Genetically Modified
Example 4011	94129	83137

The use of these codes is not mandatory, so you may not find them in all areas of the country. If your store doesn't use them, you may request this from the store owner as a courtesy to consumers.

Food Combinations

We have been taught all our lives that all the food groups can be eaten together and for some of us this works. AICR advocates the "New American Plate," which is one filled with plant-based foods like vegetables, fruits, whole grains, and beans covering two-thirds of the plate. One third or less of the plate is covered with animal protein: meat, fish, poultry, or dairy.[154] This balance of whole foods works well for many of us. However, studies have shown that specific combinations of foods can help to alleviate digestive distress, as well as encourage weight management.[155] A precise method of food combining suggests you eat or avoid eating certain groups of foods at the same time. For example, when planning a meal, combine food groups of animal protein with complex carbohydrates such as green leafy vegetables (e.g., spinach, kale, beet greens, or broccoli). Alternately, combine more starchy vegetables such as corn, potatoes, or pasta with complex carbohydrates such as a salad of green leafy vegetables and raw or cooked non-starchy vegetables like broccoli. Avoid combining proteins with high starch carbohydrates such as pasta, rice, or potatoes. Try eating fruits alone about half an hour before or after a meal. This method of food combining also promotes the body's internal cleansing process and will boost the maximizing of nutrients and minimizing of calories.[156]

Here are some suggestions for combining food groups in your own meal preparations:

Good Combinations

All green vegetables can be combined with starches.

All green vegetables can be combined with all proteins.

Poor Combinations

Avoid proteins with fruits.

Avoid proteins with starches.

Avoid starches with fruits.

If raw, high-fiber vegetables create a digestive issue for you, then try steaming or sautéing these foods.

If you have already started a program to lose weight and have reached a plateau where results are stagnant, try this method of food combining for three to four weeks. You might be surprised with the results. As you create your unique plate to support your health, habits of food combining (if this works for you) will become second nature and part of your lifestyle.

Portion Sizes

With the awareness of how food fuels the body and your development of a long-term healthy eating habit, occasional food deviations are okay. You should not feel guilty to splurge now and then if you are routinely physically active and making the food choices appropriate to your caloric needs. So, when you sample a tasty dish and yearn for a second helping, go for it!

The portion chart below can help you visualize how to balance and create your unique plate. Note the calories derived from a cup of rice or pasta versus a cup of veggies. The size of a baseball or an adult's closed fist can be a quick guide for one serving of grains, fruit, or vegetables. The length of your hand up to the wrist can be one serving of meat, fish, or poultry. You might be surprised to learn that one teaspoon or one ounce of some of your popular snacks or spreads will quickly add up the caloric content as you increase the number of teaspoons.

THE SIZE OF A	EQUIVALENT	FOODS	CALORIES
	1 cup	Rice, pasta Fruit Veggies	200 75 40
	3 ounces	Meat Fish Poultry	160 160 160
	1 ounce	Nuts Raisins	170 85
	1 ounce	Chips Popcorn Pretzels	150 120 120
	1 ounce	Peanut butter Hard cheese	170 100
	1 teaspoon	Cooking oil Mayonnaise, butter Sugar	40 35 15

© 2013 Integrative Nutrition Inc. (Used with permission.)[157]

The awareness of portion sizes and their contents can make a world of difference to your caloric intake, depending on the food. Identify your daily activity level so that you can adjust your portions when necessary. As you balance the foods on your plate and decide to increase portions, first start with vegetables, followed by greens or salads with healthy fats, and lastly animal protein and grains. If you choose to get your proteins from legumes, then you need to adjust the number of your servings and snacks accordingly. Again, this depends on the level of activity in your daily routine. Keep these portion sizes in mind whenever you eat out and, when appropriate, request a carry-out container to take home your divided, uneaten portions.

If one of your comfort meals is a breakfast that includes eggs, bacon or sausage, biscuits and gravy, you don't have to give up this pleasure. Arrange small portions on your plate (or share this meal with someone) add green vegetables and some berries to balance it.

Avoid eating to the point where you feel the need to loosen your belt. It is best to get in a habit of walking away from your plate before you feel full. Depending on your work schedule, your main meals, such as those that include grains, meats, vegetables, salad, and a dessert, should be eaten during the most active times of your daily routine so the body can utilize most of the calories and not have to store them. Allow yourself four to five hours when eating a main meal before going to bed. If you must eat close to your bedtime, focus on having something light but nourishing. My favorite nighttime snack is four to five wheat crackers with almond butter (or hummus) and a cup of chicken broth. Making these conscious changes in your eating habits can bring about amazing results if you are struggling to lose a required amount of weight.

Starting Your Day

The body undergoes a daily elimination cycle mostly carried out at night and in the early morning before awakening. This elimination cycle requires a rest of 10 to 12 hours from your last meal. If you are not getting at least six hours of restful sleep each night, focus on correcting this.

If you work a nightshift and sleep during the day, you will need to consider this in your meal planning. Breakfast is what kick-starts your metabolism and, depending on your career, family size, and activity level, you may require three regular meals a day with a few snacks in between or four to five meals with smaller portions. So, whether you find yourself rushed in the mornings or not hungry, you need to boost the body's metabolism starting with a beverage or a glass of water. Water, when consumed a half hour before meals, tends to make you feel full and will start the body's cleansing process. Later, a nutritious snack (e.g., handful of nuts, piece of fruit), a green smoothie, or sitting down to a relaxed, balanced breakfast (e.g., grains, omelet with vegetables) will enhance the start of your day.

Here is one of my favorite choices for breakfast: half a bowl of cooked oatmeal or quinoa, added to this, one half teaspoon cinnamon, one teaspoon of honey or condensed milk, and a quarter cup of kefir. I top it off with a handful of blueberries (or chopped strawberries) and a handful of chopped walnuts. Depending on my activity level, this meal will sustain me for five to six hours. Another one of my breakfast treats is an eight-ounce bowl of vegetable or chicken soup, a slice of toast covered with a tablespoon of hummus, and a handful of fresh blueberries. Whenever I yearn for an omelet, I include a variety of chopped vegetables and herbs, making it large enough to serve a second time.

You will discover that not all sugar is bad for you. The sugar found in fruit, grains, and milk is good for you. The sugar to avoid or decrease on your plate will be that found mainly in processed foods: donuts, cakes, muffins, pancake syrup, sodas, sweet teas, coffee with added sugar, and even some breakfast bars – read labels and ask questions.

The number of meals and snacks your body needs will fall into place as you experiment with combining foods and hydrating during the day. Planning and preparing your meals in advance and including quality supplements as part of your daily regimen will allow you to fuel your body appropriately. You will be surprised to discover reduced cravings.

7

Cook Once, Eat Three Times or More

Wouldn't it be convenient to be able to come home and put a balanced, nutritious meal together in 15 to 20 minutes? What makes this possible? In this chapter, I will share the method that makes this possible for me. I call it "cook once, eat three times or more." Of course, the "three times or more" will depend on your family size. This approach will not only introduce you to including more whole foods in your diet (if you are not already doing so) but also encourages an effortless way to reach your daily five or more servings of fruits and vegetables that are so important in achieving the acid–alkaline balance for the body, which in turn helps with weight management.

This approach includes planning, preparing, and cooking meals and snacks for at least three to five days in advance. Putting this plan in operation allows for the creation of nutritious on-the-go meals as well as family sit-down meals. You will save money if you tend to eat out often and, most importantly, have control of what goes into your meals. In addition, your home-cooked meals can generate a positive energy of love for those around you, an energy that is therapeutic, creates joyful memories, and contributes to the happiness of everyone in your presence.

My brother would always preface his financial advice to me with the phrase, "There is no free lunch." So, with this reality in mind, *you do need to invest some time up front to accomplish cooking once and eating three*

times or more. As you practice this method of advanced meal preparation, you may even find time two to three times a week to enjoy some activities you didn't think were possible.

You may already have recipe ideas for plant-based meals and snacks. However, if you are not familiar with this way of cooking, you will find at the end of this book, a few of my basic recipes used to prepare some of the components for my weekly meals. They allow for easy substitution of various ingredients so that you can create balanced meals for at least three to five days depending on your family size.

Growing up on the island of Trinidad (Trinidad and Tobago), I was always surrounded by fresh, whole foods including a variety of greens, vegetables, spices, and herbs. At that time, I didn't realize how **essential** these foods are in supporting a healthy body. After I learned of the benefits of nutrition from my nutritional dietary studies, my meal creations included whole foods, as often as possible.

Herbs and spices are plant based, enriched with healing properties, and have been used for centuries as part of "nature's medicine chest."[158] Not only will herbs and spices support major body systems (e.g., immune system), but they also add flavor and color that can turn a simple dish into an extraordinary, savory meal. If you are not familiar with the use of herbs and spices in cooking, get ready for an awakening experience in your meal planning.

I set aside one day a week for grocery shopping and one day for cooking and other meal preparations. Organic meats and vegetables are usually my first choice and I try to have the following herbs and spices on hand: ginger root, garlic, onions, rosemary, cilantro, oregano, basil, powdered chili pepper, cinnamon, cumin, and turmeric. I use many other herbs from time to time in different meals. I sometimes prepare my own salsa that includes a mixture of ingredients including chopped tomatoes, small pieces of jalapeno peppers or habanero peppers, lime juice, onions, salt, garlic, cumin, and cilantro. I use a small amount of this mixture to enhance soups, sauces, and dips. ***I refer to this ingredient as gourmet salsa in the section listed as Recipes.*** There are several organic mouth-watering varieties in food stores for sale. Again, you need to read the labels before making your choice. If salsa is new to you, I suggest starting with a mild gourmet salsa.

Another favorite I have on hand for quick meals is a variety of prepared and partially prepared flatbread wraps. Some are made from sprouted grain, corn (tortilla), or flour (roti). They range in diameter from six to eight inches. After purchasing the wraps, I separate them into portions for storage. I also use cabbage and lettuce leaves to create some of my wraps. I prepare and cook in advance moderate portions of grains (e.g., quinoa, rice, noodles), vegetables, meats, casserole, soup, or an occasional large crock-pot dish. I keep canned lentils on hand to incorporate into meals during times when I am unable to prepare them from scratch. I also store organic bone broth, vegetable and chicken stock, and frozen vegetables to create quick soups when I'm unable to prepare soups in advance.

Preferably, I cook the day after grocery shopping. I purchase only enough fresh fruits, and raw vegetables needed for meals and snacks within the week to avoid spoilage and will only buy more after everything is consumed.

I rinse and prepare (i.e., chop or slice) raw vegetables (e.g., carrots, cabbage, onions, cauliflower, celery) for the first three days. Once these are consumed, I prepare more for the next three to four days. If you decide to experiment with 'food combining,' (recall Chapter 4), having these items ready ahead of time will be extremely helpful for you to stick to the food combination that works best for you. After preparing my cooked and raw food portions, I freeze or refrigerate them in storage containers with tight-fitting lids. Each week, my meal creations vary by what items are on sale and what fruits and vegetables are in season.

I prefer to marinate my chicken, fish, or meat overnight (preferably the night before cooking) to achieve maximum flavor. The necessary ingredients for casserole and stove-top dishes are prepped and presorted the night before, which allows meals to be completed sooner the following day.

I utilize two timers at the beginning of my baking session. Once the oven is heated (on cooking day), I bake fish, roast vegetables, bake/roast one or two chickens, and a casserole. I first insert the vegetables to be roasted and the chicken(s) to be baked/roasted. The roasted vegetables take less time to cook, so once I remove them from the oven, the casserole is next inserted as the chicken continues to bake/roast. If there is sufficient space left in the oven, fish to be baked can also be inserted at this time. As these items are baking, I start the preparation for stove top cooking. This might be a large portion of vegetable soup or a crock-pot meal. Grains and lentils may be also cooked during this time. ***I emphasize, when trying this method of advanced food preparation, start with two preparations*** (e.g., chicken and roasted vegetables, or soup and grains). Then, eventually add other preparations as you see fit.

Quinoa is frequently included in my food planning because it is a versatile and healthy grain that cooks in a short period of time. I cook it in large amounts and sometimes serve it as a breakfast cereal in place of oatmeal or add it into omelets with chopped green onions, grated carrots, and a sprinkle of chili pepper and cumin. I occasionally serve quinoa again at dinner mixed in with lentils or roasted vegetables or simply as a side dish. It works well as one of the add-in ingredients in a cabbage or lettuce wrap.

Once all the cooking is done and the food is cooled off, I divide it into labeled portions for storage. I then ***refrigerate*** two to three days' worth of portions for immediate use and freeze the rest for later use. The precooked meats and prepared vegetables become part of meals and snacks that may be combined with green salads or taken with fruit when on the run. Portions of the cooked dishes are often the main ingredients used in creating wraps. You will be amazed at the wide variety of wrap sandwiches you can create when you have a varied assortment of prepared foods available.

Hummus and avocado dips are usually my choice of spreads for my wraps, sandwiches, and raw vegetables. These balanced meals are put together in a short time for either breakfast, lunch, or dinner. Smoothies made from vegetables and fruits are sometimes substituted for a meal and these too, can be prepared quickly because of the availability of chopped vegetables. A salad of either lettuce or spinach (or both), grated carrots, sliced avocado, sliced apples, dried cranberries, and pumpkin seeds is one example that I create and store for a day or two to complete my dinners.

Foods such as muffins, breads, or cakes are prepared at other convenient times or carefully selected as part of my shopping list when needed. These too, are proportioned, refrigerated, or stored in the freezer to serve with future meals or used as snacks. A must on my shopping list is a variety of pickled vegetables that are added to enhance my wraps and snacks.

During the preparation and cooking of my meals, I always have my favorite music playing in the background and many times I enjoy a glass of wine. If you decide to experiment with this method of meal planning, try to encourage other members of your household to participate. You can find simple tasks for everyone. Making this a part of your family time will benefit all involved, knowing they are participating in the preparations of their meals. It can also create conversations and learning moments. You will be amazed to discover how much fun this activity can be.

If you decide to experiment with this method of advanced food preparations, first start the baking process by planning two dishes, then, once you are comfortable and have become more adept with preparing two dishes, plan to add another the next time. Do likewise for the preparation and cooking of stove-top meals.

As you begin to incorporate portions from the different food groups in your meals, you will be able to decrease your animal protein intake, which is good for your body and your checkbook. You may even want to experiment with some meatless meals. However, before you do, start by decreasing your portion size of meats (e.g., chicken, beef, fish). Then, try replacing meat with vegetable dishes once a week. As your body adjusts to the changes, you may find it easier to eat less animal protein or omit them from most of your meals. Your activity level will be key to making the necessary adjustments as you experiment with portion sizes and different food groups.

With this approach to food planning, putting together a variety of meals and salads or packing one to take with you becomes automatic when the fixings are readily available. The recipes I have shared with you in the Recipe section of this book, serve as a foundation for you to create your own dishes.

8

Connect the Pieces

You might already be aware of the ample amount of health information readily available via the internet, fitness magazines, health books, and even from your own physician. What obstacles prevent you from owning and making your health a top priority? Let's face it, aging is inevitable, and the chances of developing diseases increase with age. Can you think of five things you should be doing for your health, but you are not currently doing? I believe that as you journey through life connecting your health pieces, you can achieve the benefits of amazing health despite challenges and obstacles. Your unique pathway will emerge, and age will become just a number. Your involvement in managing your health along this journey will be the beginning of slowing down the aging process, and your positive results will be the fulfilling feedback to nurture your mind, body, and soul.

I use the circle of life exercise as my umbrella to keep me in check and have deduced five health actions I would like to share with you, as I conclude this section of the book. After trying these, you can modify or add to them to fit your specific needs based on your results. Remember, you are unique and can be in control of your amazing body. ***Action*** is important for any change to take place in your life and yes, also being ***consistent*** and ***disciplined.***

Action 1: Get an Annual Wellness Screen

Make this a priority. Even if you "feel well," it is safer to go further to know your health status with a wellness screen. Know the cost of this assessment ahead of time. Include this expenditure in your financial planning to make it possible whether it is covered by health insurance or not. If you do not already have a primary care doctor, get one.

Know Your Numbers For:
- Blood pressure
- Waist Circumference/BMI
- Fasting Glucose
- HDL cholesterol
- Triglycerides
- Hemoglobin
- Vitamin D
- Glycated Hemoglobin (Hemoglobin A1C- when applicable)

Action 2: Schedule Physical Activity

Include physical activity in your busy schedule. If exercise is not part of your lifestyle, start with at least one activity or exercise two to three times a week. This might include brisk walking, dancing, or a walk-run jog for 20 to 30 minutes. Increase the number of activities or exercises you do per week as you develop this habit. The benefits gained from physical exercise are ***enormous.***

Action 3: Plan and Prepare Meals

Plan and prepare at least three to five days of meals and snacks in advance. Include whole, heart-healthy foods and have a shopping list ready before you head off to the supermarket.

Action 4: Schedule Enjoyable Activities

Schedule an enjoyable activity for yourself, or with family or a friend, at least once a week. This may include a picnic, gardening, watching a movie, experimenting with a new recipe, or attending an event or lecture that will entertain or educate. The emotional benefits to be derived from this habit in your life are **priceless**.

Action 5: Develop a Self-Care Strategy

Develop a self-care strategy to help you when you feel overwhelmed or stressed. Include a list of trustworthy people with whom you can talk. Volunteer and prove to be a trustworthy person yourself to relatives, friends and even charitable and supportive foundations.

It is well worth the time and diligence to discover your unique approach to **diet and supplementation, exercise, stress reduction, and health preventive measures.** As you connect these health pieces, you will realize that having the tools on hand will help to create habits with positive outcomes. This will reinforce your motivation and will allow you to return to your healthy path, whenever you waver. Be on the lookout for more scientific discoveries to help you stay on this track. Are you ready to become the best "you" you can be?

"And will you succeed?
Yes! You Will, indeed!
(98 and ¾ percent guaranteed.)"
—Dr. Seuss [159]

Recipes - Let's Start Cooking

The recipes I share with you here are the basic ones I utilize to "Cook Once, Eat Three Times or More," as described in Chapter 7. These recipes provide the components for many of my weekly meals and snacks which I put together within 15 to 20 minutes. However, you will need to spend some time up front to prepare them so that portions can be added to wraps, salads, as well as used as part of a balanced meal. Remember your goal here is to reach your daily five or more servings of fruits and vegetables. Your family size will determine how long these meals will last.

Cooking can be fun as well as healing, once you decide to take control of your health and the ingredients are readily available. Preparation is essential, as seen in all aspects of life, and that fact carries over if you decide to experiment with this approach. I stress, start with preparing two meals in advance, then add more as you go along. Get ready to enjoy a new eating experience!

- Multi-Use Marinade (to be used with chicken, fish, or beef)
- Creamy Sweet Potato and Garbanzo Soup (without the cream)
- Baked/Roasted Chicken (or Fish)
- Angela's Peppy Hummus
- Baked/ Roasted Vegetables
- Get Up and Go Smoothie (sometimes used as a meal replacement.)
- All-Purpose Vinaigrette Salad Dressing

Temperatures may vary with different ovens. So, as you try these recipes you can adjust your oven temperature accordingly. Coconut oil is solid at room temperature, a couple of seconds in the microwave will liquefy it. The gourmet salsa included in some of the recipes is optional.

These recipes can be easily modified by substituting different vegetables, meats, herbs, and spices.

Multi-Use Marinade

Ingredients

Juice squeezed from 2 medium limes or 1 large lime

4–6 crushed garlic cloves

1/2–3/4 teaspoon sea salt (depending on quantity of chicken and personal preference)

1/4 teaspoon chili pepper powder or 2 tablespoons gourmet salsa*

* Optional ingredient, but I encourage you to try it at least once.

Directions

Mix the ingredients above in a small glass bowl until blended and then set aside or refrigerate for later use.

Creamy Sweet Potato and Garbanzo Soup
(without the cream)

This recipe requires a large pot and blender. It is one of my favorite soups because it provides a boost of energy any time of the day.

Ingredients

29 oz. can garbanzos, drained

3 medium-sized or 2 large baked, sweet potatoes (can be baked in the microwave), cooled and cut into chunks

32 oz. broth of any kind (e.g., chicken, vegetable, or bone)

3–3½ cups water

1½ inch piece fresh ginger root, sliced

1 large onion or two medium onions, sliced

3/4–1 teaspoon sea salt

5 crushed garlic cloves

1–2 teaspoons gourmet salsa*

2½ tablespoons coconut oil (approximately)

3–4 tablespoons finely chopped cilantro or mint leaves for garnish.

Directions

Heat coconut oil in a frying pan on a low flame. Add crushed garlic and sauté for two to three minutes. Add sliced onions, mix in and sauté for an additional three to four minutes. Add sliced ginger, mix in and sauté for three more minutes and then set aside.

In a blender, add one cup of water and one cup broth along with portions of garbanzos, sweet potato, and some of the sautéed onion mixture. Liquefy for 30 seconds and then pour into a large pot. Continue to blend portions of garbanzos, sweet potatoes, and onion mixture. Liquefy, and continue this process until all ingredients have been blended and added to the pot.

Add salt, mix well, and bring to a boil, while stirring occasionally. Cover and let simmer on a low heat for 10 to 12 minutes. The goal is to achieve a not-too-thick consistency. Add additional water if it becomes too thick. Just before removing from the heat, add gourmet salsa, and mix in. Allow soup to cool before proportioning for storage. Store refrigerated portions for the next two days or freeze portions for later use. Garnish with chopped cilantro or mint leaves.

Baked/Roasted Chicken (or Fish)

The multi-use marinade is used with this recipe. Whole or cut-up chicken, fish (e.g., salmon, tilapia, cod) or even a pot roast might be marinated overnight with this mixture).

Directions for Baking/Roasting Chicken

Before marinating the whole chicken, remove the giblets and any visible fat under and around the skin areas. Thoroughly rinse the inside and outside of the chicken and let it drain completely. With your fingers, gently loosen the skin over the breast, thighs, and back of the chicken. Use a knife to make small slits in areas where the skin is difficult to loosen.

Place the well-drained chicken in a roasting pan or dish. Use your fingers to spread the prepared marinade inside the chicken cavity and in and around the loosened skin. If you find most of the marinade is used up before spreading all over the chicken, prepare an additional half of the marinade ingredients to complete the process and make note for future reference. Wash your hands immediately after this procedure. Place the chicken breast-side down, cover the pan or dish tightly with foil, and refrigerate overnight or for one to two hours. The longer you marinate the more flavorful the outcome.

Just before baking/roasting the chicken, put together the following ingredients in a small bowl to form a paste and set aside. This preparation is optional. But when used the outcome is more appetizing.

Ingredients

2 tablespoons fresh minced rosemary or 3 teaspoons dried rosemary

1½ tablespoons coconut oil (first bring to liquid)

1/2 teaspoon ground clove

1/2 teaspoon cumin powder

1 small lime, cut in half (Optional, to be used after carving)

Preheat oven to 375°F.

The total baking time for four to five pounds of chicken is approximately 60 to 70 minutes.

Remove the foil and drain the juices from the marinated chicken. With your fingers, distribute the above paste mixture in the cavity and under and over the entire loosened skin areas. Make sure the chicken is positioned breast-side down and that the pan is tightly covered with foil. Place the chicken in the oven to bake for approximately 45 to 50 minutes. After this period, remove the chicken from the oven, carefully remove the foil (save for later use), turn the chicken breast-side up, and return to oven. Allow to roast for 15 to 20 minutes until chicken is golden brown, the skin recedes from the thigh bones and the liquids run clear when pierced with a sharp knife. You will notice some liquids collected in the pan, which you should save for later use.

Remove the chicken from the oven, cover with foil, and let sit for 5-10 minutes before carving. Squeeze the juice of the small lime over the carved chicken and re-cover tightly.

I sometimes use portions of the baked/roasted chicken to create a balanced meal, and portions are stored for later use in wraps, salads or added to raw vegetables. Again, your family size will determine how long this will last. Some of the liquids collected from the final roasting process can be drizzled sparingly (since most of the chicken fat is present) over the ready-to-eat portions. To remove most of the fat from the liquid portion, pour into a glass container, allow to cool to room temperature, cover and refrigerate two to three hours (or overnight). Most of the fat will rise to the surface as the liquid cools and you can remove it. The liquid portion will appear gelled. This is nutritious and flavorful. It can be used to make gravy, to flavor sautéed vegetables, to cook with lentils, or to add to soups. Before freezing or refrigerating cooked chicken portions, add in some of this jelled liquid.

Directions for Baking/ Roasting Fish

When preparing fresh fish, rinse well and pat dry with paper towel. For frozen fish, allow to thaw according to the directions, rinse and pat dry with paper towel. Place in a glass baking dish with the overnight Multi-Use marinade mixture and cover tightly with foil. The multi-use marinade will serve well for two to three pounds of fish. If less, use half the ingredients for marinade. Marinate over night or for 2- 3 hours before baking. The longer the marinating the more flavorful the outcome.

Preheat the oven to 375°F.

Have ready 1 ½ tablespoons coconut oil

Before baking, mix the following ingredients together in a small bowl:

- 1 teaspoon ground clove
- 1/2 teaspoon coriander or cumin powder (or a mixture of both)

Pour off the marinate juices before baking. Sprinkle the clove and coriander/cumin mixture over the fish then drizzle with coconut oil. Cover with foil and bake for 12-15 minutes. Remove foil, and roast, uncovered for 8-10 minutes or until fish flakes when pierced with a fork. Remove from oven, cover tightly, allow to cool if you plan to refrigerate for later use.

Angela's Peppy Hummus

This dip can be used with wraps or on steamed or raw vegetables.

Ingredients

Juice squeezed from 1 medium lime

15 oz. can chickpeas/garbanzos (do not drain)

½ cup tahini

1 tablespoon olive oil

1 tablespoon minced garlic

½ tablespoon salt (or adjust to taste)

½–1 tablespoon gourmet salsa*(optional)

2 tablespoons cilantro, finely chopped

Directions

Blend the chickpeas with the tahini in a food processor or blender on low speed. Transfer to a glass bowl and add in olive oil, lime juice, garlic, salt, salsa, and mix well. Just before serving garnish with cilantro. This can last 3-4 days (depending on family size) when covered tightly and kept refrigerated.

Baked / Roasted Vegetables

Any hard-textured vegetables can be used for this recipe. Removing the skin of the hard-textured vegetables will allow a shorter time for baking/roasting but is not required.

Preheat oven to 425°F.

Ingredients

2 medium carrots, cut into moderate chunks

1½ cups brussel sprouts cut into halves (depending on size) OR 1 small cauliflower head, broken into large chunks

1 of each bell pepper (green, yellow, and red), cut into large chunks

1 large sweet potato, cut into chunks

1 large onion, cut into large chunks

1 small, hard-textured pumpkin, cut into chunks

2½ tablespoons coconut oil

1 teaspoon sea salt

½ teaspoon fresh ground black pepper

¼ teaspoon chili powder (optional)

1½ teaspoons coriander or cumin powder (or a mixture of both)

Directions

Before chopping, rinse all vegetables in cold water, drain well. While draining, mix together salt, black pepper, chili powder, and coriander mixture in a small bowl, set aside.

Place brussels sprouts and chopped vegetables into a large resealable, plastic, storage bag. (Depending on the size of the resealable bag, the following process to coat the vegetables with oil may have to be repeated). Drizzle the coconut oil intermittently over the chopped vegetables in the storage bag. Close tightly, shake and mix well to coat the vegetables until all the oil has been poured into the bag. Spread one layer of the coated vegetables in a large, shallow baking dish. Lightly sprinkle the salt/pepper/herb mixture over the vegetables. Cover dish with foil and bake for 18 to 20 minutes. Remove the foil and roast for an additional five to eight minutes or until the vegetables feel slightly tender when pierced with a fork. Remove dish from oven and allow to cool, if for future storage.

These tasty vegetables can be used as a side dish, added to wraps, mixed in with greens, or folded into an omelet.

Get Up and Go Smoothie

This smoothie can be a replacement meal or a post-workout snack.

Ingredients

10 oz. almond or coconut milk (add more milk to adjust consistency to your desire)

½ cup mixed greens

1 scoop protein powder (vegan)

½ avocado

½ cup ripe, frozen mango chunks (frozen pineapple or banana can be substituted.)

¼ cup ice cubes

Directions

Combine all the above ingredients in a blender and liquefy until smooth. Enjoy!

All-Purpose Vinaigrette Salad Dressing

This vinaigrette dressing is appetizing on salads, cooked chicken, fish, or steamed vegetables, and can be included in wraps.

Ingredients

1½ teaspoon Dijon mustard
1-2 teaspoons apple cider vinegar (or adjust to taste)
2 tablespoons olive oil
1–2 tablespoons lemon juice (adjust to taste)
1 teaspoon finely chopped onions
½ teaspoon sea salt (or adjust to taste)
1¼ tablespoons honey or maple syrup

Directions

In a small bowl, whisk together the lemon juice, apple cider vinegar, mustard, and honey. While whisking, slowly add in oil. Add chopped onions, salt, and mix well. Refrigerate the dressing in a glass jar with tight fitting lid.

If this is all new to you, experiment with these dishes and substitute some of your favorite vegetables. Remember it is never too late to get on a healthy path. Only you can be in control of your personal health.

Helpful Websites

www.healthgrades.com

www.aicr.org

www.integrativenutrition.com

www.LifeExtension.com

www.cdc.gov

If you live in Illinois, http://insurance.illinois.gov

www.SpectraCell.com

www.fda.gov/Food/www.aicr.org/can-prevent/healthy-recipes

www.acefitness.org/acefit/fitness-facts

www.growingstronger.nutrition.tufts.edu

References

1. Dr. Seuss, *Oh, The Places You'll Go!* (London: Harper Collins, 2003), 2.

2. Life Extension, *Disease Prevention and Treatment,* 5th ed. (Fort Lauderdale, FL: Life Extension Publications, 2013), 789.

3. Lyle MacWilliam, *NutriSearch Comparative Guide to Nutritional Supplements,* (Kelowna, BC: Northern Dimensions Publishing, 2014), 7-9.

4. "Definitions," Health Promotion Advocates, last modified June 14, 2011, healthpromotionadvocates.org/historical-reference/definitions/.

5. Catherine Sheehan. Clinical *Immunology Principles and Laboratory Diagnosis,* 2nd ed. (Philadelphia, PA: Lippincott-Raven Publishers, 1997), 3, 14.

6. Elizabeth Lipski, Digestive Wellness: *Strengthen the Immune System and Prevent Disease Through Healthy Digestion,* 4th ed. (New York, NY: McGraw-Hill Education, 2012), 10, 51.

7. World Cancer Research Fund and American Institute for Cancer Research, F*ood, Nutrition, Physical Activity, and the Prevention of Cancer: A Global Perspective* (Washington DC: AICR, 2007), 38.

8. Elizabeth Lipski, *Digestive Wellness: Strengthen the Immune System and Prevent Disease Through Healthy Digestion,* 4th ed. (New York, NY: McGraw-Hill Education, 2012), 90.

9*. Life Extension,* Disease Prevention and Treatment, 5th ed. (Fort Lauderdale, FL: Life Extension Publications, 2013), 164.

10. "Heart Disease and Stroke Statistics 2018 At-a-Glance," American Heart Association /American Stroke Association, life is why, accessed June 2018, https://healthmetrics.heart.org/wp-content/uploads/2018/02/At-A-Glance.

11. "Heart Disease and Stroke Statistics 2018 At-a-Glance," American Heart Association /American Stroke Association, life is why, accessed June 2018, https://healthmetrics.heart.org/wp-content/uploads/2018/02/At-A-Glance.

12. "Heart Disease and Stroke Statistics 2018 At-A-Glance," American Heart

Association/American Stroke Association, life is why, accessed June 2018. https://healthmetrics.heart.org/wp-content/uploads/2018/02/At-A-Glance.

13. "Heart Disease and Stroke Statistics 2018 At-A-Glance," American Heart Association/American Stroke Association, life is why, accessed June 2018. https://healthmetrics.heart.org/wp-content/uploads/2018/02/At-A-Glance.

14. "Heart Disease and Stroke Statistics 2018 At-A-Glance," American Heart Association/American Stroke Association, life is why, accessed June 2018. https://healthmetrics.heart.org/wp-content/uploads/2018/02/At-A-Glance.

15. "Heart Disease and Stroke Statistics 2018 At-A-Glance," American Heart Association/American Stroke Association, life is why, accessed June 2018. https://healthmetrics.heart.org/wp-content/uploads/2018/02/At-A-Glance.

16. "Heart Disease and Stroke Statistics 2018 At-A-Glance," American Heart Association/American Stroke Association, life is why, accessed June 2018. https://healthmetrics.heart.org/wp-content/uploads/2018/02/At-A-Glance.

17. Elizabeth Lipski, *Digestive Wellness: Strengthen the Immune System and Prevent Disease Through Healthy Digestion,* 4th ed. (New York, NY: McGraw-Hill Education, 2012), 382.

18. "About Metabolic Syndrome," accessed May 2018. www.heart.org/HEARTORG/Conditions/More/MetabolicSyndrome/About-Metabolic-Syndrome_UCM_301920_Article.jsp.

19. "Heart Disease and Stroke Statistics 2018 At-A-Glance," American Heart Association/American Stroke Association, life is why, accessed June 2018. https://healthmetrics.heart.org/wp-content/uploads/2018/02/At-A-Glance.

20. World Cancer Research Fund/American Institute for Cancer Research. Food, Nutrition, Physical Activity, and the Prevention of Cancer: A Global Perspective (Washington, DC: AICR, 2007), 40.

21. Elizabeth Lipski, *Digestive Wellness: Strengthen the Immune System and Prevent Disease Through Healthy Digestion,* 4th ed. (New York, NY: McGraw-Hill Education, 2012), 255.

22. Elizabeth Lipski, *Digestive Wellness: Strengthen the Immune System and Prevent Disease Through Healthy Digestion,* 4th ed. (New York, NY: McGraw-Hill Education, 2012), 251

23. Catherine Sheehan, *Clinical Immunology Principles and Laboratory Diagnosis,* 2nd ed. (Philadelphia, PA: Lippincott-Raven Publishers, 1997), 4.

24. "Heart Disease and Stroke Statistics 2018 At-A-Glance," American Heart Association/American Stroke Association, life is why, accessed June 2018. https://healthmetrics.heart.org/wp-content/uploads/2018/02/At-A-Glance.

25. Life Extension Life Extension, *Disease Prevention and Treatment,* 5th ed. (Fort Lauderdale, FL: Life Extension Publications, 2013), 1074–75.

26. "Health screening," faqs.org, accessed May 18, 2015. www.faqs.org/health/topics/72/Health-screening.html.

27. "Health screening," faqs.org, accessed May 18, 2015. www.faqs.org/health/topics/72/Health-screening.html.

28. Life Extension, *Disease Prevention and Treatment,* 5th ed. (Fort Lauderdale, FL: Life Extension Publications, 2013), 745-746.

29. Life Extension, *Disease Prevention and Treatment,* 5th ed. (Fort Lauderdale, FL: Life Extension Publications, 2013), 745.

30. World Cancer Research Fund and American Institute for Cancer Research. *Food, Nutrition, Physical Activity, and the Prevention of Cancer: A Global Perspective* (Washington, DC: AICR, 2007), 212.

31. World Cancer Research Fund and American Institute for Cancer Research. *Food, Nutrition, Physical Activity, and the Prevention of Cancer: A Global Perspective* (Washington, DC: AICR, 2007), 212.

32. World Cancer Research Fund and American Institute for Cancer Research. *Food, Nutrition, Physical Activity, and the Prevention of Cancer: A Global Perspective* (Washington, DC: AICR, 2007), 212.

33. "About Metabolic Syndrome," accessed June 2018. www.heart.org/HEARTORG/Conditions/More/MetabolicSyndrome/About-Metabolic-Syndrome_UCM_301920_Article.jsp.

34. Richard Ravel, *Clinical Laboratory Medicine,* 6th ed. (St. Louis, MO: Mosby, 1995), 3.

35. Michael L. Bishop et al, *Clinical Chemistry, Principles, Procedures, Correlations,* 4th ed. (Philadelphia, PA: Lippincott Williams & Wilkins, 2000), 22.

36. Life Extension, *Disease Prevention and Treatment,* 5th ed. (Fort Lauderdale, FL: Life Extension Publications, 2013), 220.

37. Life Extension, *Disease Prevention and Treatment,* 5th ed. (Fort Lauderdale, FL: Life Extension Publications, 2013), 220-225

38. Life Extension, *Disease Prevention and Treatment,* 5th ed. (Fort Lauderdale, FL: Life Extension Publications, 2013), 225.

39. Life Extension, *Disease Prevention and Treatment,* 5th ed. (Fort Lauderdale, FL: Life Extension Publications, 2013), 437-438.

40. Life Extension, *Disease Prevention and Treatment,*5th ed. (Fort Lauderdale, FL: Life Extension Publications, 2013), 221.

41. Life Extension, *Disease Prevention and Treatment,* 5th ed. (Fort Lauderdale, FL: Life Extension Publications, 2013), 221.

42. Life Extension, *Disease Prevention and Treatment,* 5th ed. (Fort Lauderdale, FL: Life Extension Publications, 2013), 437.

43. Life Extension, *Disease Prevention and Treatment,* 5th ed. (Fort Lauderdale, FL: Life Extension Publications, 2013), 221.

44. Life Extension, *Disease Prevention and Treatment,* 5th ed. (Fort Lauderdale, FL: Life Extension Publications, 2013), 221.

45. Life Extension, *Disease Prevention and Treatment,* 5th ed. (Fort Lauderdale, FL: Life Extension Publications, 2013), 221.

46. Lyle MacWilliam, *NutriSearch Comparative Guide to Nutritional Supplements,* 5th ed. (Kelowna, BC: Northern Dimensions Publishing, 2014), 19-28.

47. Life Extension, *Disease Prevention and Treatment,* 5th ed. (Fort Lauderdale, FL: Life Extension Publications, 2013), 230.

48. Elizabeth Lipski, *Digestive Wellness: Strengthen the Immune System and Prevent Disease Through Healthy Digestion,* 4th ed. (New York, NY: McGraw-Hill Education, 2012), 251-252.

49. Michael L. Bishop et al, *Clinical Chemistry, Principles, Procedures, Correlations,* 4th ed. (Philadelphia, PA: Lippincott Williams & Wilkins, 2000), 294.

50. "About Metabolic Syndrome," accessed May 2018. www.heart.org/HEARTORG/Conditions/More/MetabolicSyndrome/About-Metabolic-Syndrome_UCM_301920_Article.jsp.

51. Life Extension, *Disease Prevention and Treatment,* 5th ed. (Fort Lauderdale, FL: Life Extension Publications, 2013), 437.

52. Life Extension, *Disease Prevention and Treatment,* 5th ed. (Fort Lauderdale, FL: Life Extension Publications, 2013), 222.

53. Life Extension, *Disease Prevention and Treatment,* 5th ed. (Fort Lauderdale, FL: Life Extension Publications, 2013), 539.

54. Lyle MacWilliam, *NutriSearch Comparative Guide to Nutritional Supplements,* 5th ed. (Kelowna, BC: Northern Dimensions Publishing, 2014), 63.

55. Lyle MacWilliam, *NutriSearch Comparative Guide to Nutritional Supplements,* 5th ed. (Kelowna, BC: Northern Dimensions Publishing, 2014), 32.

56. "Micronutrient Test Panel" SpectraCell Laboratory, accessed March 2002, https://www.spectracell.com/micronutrient-test-panel.

57. "Micronutrient Test Panel" SpectraCell Laboratory, accessed March 2002, https://www.spectracell.com/micronutrient-test-panel.

58. American Institute for Cancer Research, *The New American Plate®: Meals for a Healthy Weight and a Healthy Life.* (Washington, D.C.: AICR Publications, E4B-NAP November 2014), 5–9.

59. American Institute for Cancer Research, *More Food, Fewer Calories: The Science of Calorie Density,* (Washington, D.C.: AICR Publications, E38-CD August 2013), 6–8.

60. American Institute for Cancer Research, *The New American Plate Veggies: Recipes for a healthy weight and a healthy life,* (Washington, D.C.: AICR Publications, E54-VEG May 2005), 3.

61. American Institute for Cancer Research, *More Food, Fewer Calories: The Science of Calorie Density,* (Washington, D.C.: AICR Publications, E38-CD August 2013), 5.

62. Joy Bauer, "Understanding the Distinction between the Caloric Density of Packaged Foods" (lecture, Institute for Integrative Nutrition, Health Coach Training Curriculum course, module 11, 2013).

63. American Institute for Cancer Research, *The AICR Guide to the Nutrition Facts Label*. (Washington, DC. AICR Publications), E2A-NF 1.

64. American Institute for Cancer Research, *The AICR Guide to the Nutrition Facts Label*. (Washington, DC. AICR Publications, E2A-NF). 3.

65. American Institute for Cancer Research, *The AICR Guide to the Nutrition Facts Label*. (Washington, DC. AICR Publications, E2A-NF). 1.

66. American Institute for Cancer Research, *The AICR Guide to the Nutrition Facts Label*. (Washington, DC. AICR Publications, E2A-NF). 3.

67. American Institute for Cancer Research, *The AICR Guide to the Nutrition Facts Label*.. (Washington, DC. AICR Publications, E2A-NF). 7.

68. Elizabeth Lipski, *Digestive Wellness: Strengthen the Immune System and Prevent Disease Through Healthy Digestion*, 4th ed. (New York, NY: McGraw-Hill Education, 2011), 140.

69. American Institute for Cancer Research, *The AICR Guide to the Nutrition Facts Label*. (Washington, DC. AICR Publications, E2A-NF). 10.

70. "Do Bodybuilders and Other Weightlifters Need More Protein?" Go Ask Alice! (accessed February 2014), http://goaskalice.columbia.edu/answered- questions/do-bodybuilders-and- other-weightlifters-need-more-protein.

71. American Institute for Cancer Research, *The AICR Guide to the Nutrition Facts Label*. (Washington, DC. AICR Publications, E2A-NF). 12.

72. American Institute for Cancer Research, *The AICR Guide to the Nutrition Facts Label*. (Washington, DC. AICR Publications, E2A-NF). 12.

73. "Changes to the Nutrition Facts Label", Food Guidance Documents, U.S. Food and Drug Administration. https:// www.fda.gov/Food/GuidanceRegulation/highlights /label.

74. "Changes to the Nutrition Facts Label", Food Guidance Documents, U.S. Food and Drug Administration. https:// www.fda.gov/Food/GuidanceRegulation/ highlights /label.

75. Ron Kennedy, "Short History of Vitamins," The Doctors' Medical Library, (accessed March 2018), 1 http://www.medical-library.net/short-history-of-vitamins/.

76. American Institute for Cancer Research, *Moving Toward a Plant-Based Diet: Menus and Recipes for Cancer Prevention Healthy Living and Lower Cancer Risk* (Washington, DC. AICR Publications, November 2001), E1B-PBD/F41, 5.

77. American Institute for Cancer Research, *Moving Toward a Plant-Based Diet: Menus and Recipes for Cancer Prevention Healthy Living and Lower Cancer Risk* (Washington, DC. AICR Publications, November 2001), E1B-PBD/F41, 5.

78. American Institute for Cancer Research, *Moving Toward a Plant-Based Diet: Menus and Recipes for Cancer Prevention Healthy Living and Lower Cancer Risk* (Washington, DC. AICR Publications, November 2001), E1B-PBD/F41, 5.

79. Jeff Primack, *Conquering Any Disease: The Ultimate High-Phytochemical Food Healing System* (Florida: Press ON Qi productions, 2012), 46.

80. Lyle MacWilliam, *NutriSearch Comparative Guide to Nutritional Supplements*, 5th ed. (Kelowna, BC: Northern Dimensions Publishing, 2014), 7.

81. Ori Hofmekler, "Metabolic Mystery Tour," *Experience Life* (November 2001): https://experiencelife.com/article/metabolic-mystery-tour/

82. Ori Hofmekler, "Metabolic Mystery Tour," *Experience Life* (November 2001): https://experiencelife.com/article/metabolic-mystery-tour/

83. "Calcium the MOST abundant mineral in the body!" SpectraCell Laboratory, (accessed March 2014), https://info.spectracell.com/bid/101803/Calcium-the-MOST-abundant-mineral-in-the-body

84. Lyle MacWilliam, *NutriSearch Comparative Guide to Nutritional Supplements*, 5th ed. (Kelowna, BC: Northern Dimensions Publishing, 2014), 29–43.

85. Elizabeth Lipski, *Digestive Wellness: Strengthen the Immune System and Prevent Disease Through Healthy Digestion*, 4th ed. (New York, NY: McGraw-Hill Education, 2011), 314.

86. American Institute for Cancer Research, *Moving Toward a Plant-Based Diet: Menus and Recipes for Cancer Prevention Healthy Living and Lower Cancer Risk* (Washington, DC. AICR Publications, November 2001), E1B-PBD/F41, 5.

87. American Institute for Cancer Research, *More Food, Fewer Calories: The Science of Calorie Density.* (Washington, DC. AICR Publications, E38-CD August 2013). 3.

88. "Do Bodybuilders and Other Weightlifters Need More Protein?" Go Ask Alice! (accessed February 2014, http://goaskalice.columbia.edu/answered-questions/do-bodybuilders-and-other-weightlifters-need-more-protein

89. Life Extension, *Disease Prevention and Treatment,* 5th ed. Fort Lauderdale, FL: Life Extension Publications, 2013), 773.

90. Paul Pitchford, *Healing with Whole Foods: Asian Traditions and Modern Nutrition,* 3rd ed. (Berkeley, CA: North Atlantic Books, 2002), 158-187

91. Life Extension, *Disease Prevention and Treatment,* 5th ed. (Fort Lauderdale, FL: Life Extension Publications, 2013), 438.

92. Jeff Primack, *Conquering Any Disease: The Ultimate High-Phytochemical Food-Healing System,* (Florida: Press ON QI productions, 2012), 157–159.

93. Jeff Primack, *Conquering Any Disease: The Ultimate High-Phytochemical Food-Healing System,* (Florida: Press ON QI productions, 2012), 158.

94. Paul Pitchford, *Healing with Whole Foods: Asian Traditions and Modern Nutrition,* 3rd ed. (Berkeley, CA: North Atlantic Books, 2002), 179.

95. Paul Pitchford, *Healing with Whole Foods: Asian Traditions and Modern Nutrition,* 3rd ed. (Berkeley, CA: North Atlantic Books, 2002), 172.

96. Paul Pitchford, *Healing with Whole Foods: Asian Traditions and Modern Nutrition,* 3rd ed. (Berkeley, CA: North Atlantic Books, 2002), 169.

97. Artemis P. Simopoulos, *Evolutionary Aspects of Diet: The Omega-6/Omega-3 Ratio and the Brain,* (Molecular Neurology January 29, 2011, [epub]

98. Paul Pitchford, *Healing with Whole Foods: Asian Traditions and Modern Nutrition,* 3rd ed. (Berkeley, CA: North Atlantic Books, 2002), 181–182.

99. Paul Pitchford, *Healing with Whole Foods: Asian Traditions and Modern Nutrition,* 3rd ed. (Berkeley, CA: North Atlantic Books, 2002), 181.

100. "Trans Fats Banned in NYC Restaurants," Harvard Health Publishing, last modified March 2007, https://www.health.harvard.edu/family-health-guide/trans-fats-banned-in-nyc-restaurants.

101. Jeff Primack, *Conquering Any Disease: The Ultimate High-Phytochemical Food-Healing System,* (Florida: Press ON QI productions, 2012), 159.

102. Elizabeth Lipski, *Digestive Wellness: Strengthen the Immune System and Prevent Disease Through Healthy Digestion,* 4th ed. (New York, NY: McGraw-Hill Education, 2011), 141.

103. Elizabeth Lipski, *Digestive Wellness: Strengthen the Immune System and Prevent Disease Through Healthy Digestion,* 4th ed. (New York, NY: McGraw-Hill Education, 2011), 280.

104. Elizabeth Lipski, *Digestive Wellness: Strengthen the Immune System and Prevent Disease Through Healthy Digestion,* 4th ed. (New York, NY: McGraw-Hill Education, 2011), 140.

105. Elizabeth Lipski, *Digestive Wellness: Strengthen the Immune System and Prevent Disease Through Healthy Digestion,* 4th ed. (New York, NY: McGraw-Hill Education, 2011), 140.

106. American Institute for Cancer Research, *The New American Plate: Meals For A Healthy Weight And A Healthy Life,* (Washington, DC. AICR Publications, E4B-NAP, updated November 2014). 3.

107. Lyle MacWilliam, *NutriSearch Comparative Guide to Nutritional Supplements,* 5th ed. (Kelowna, BC: Northern Dimensions Publishing, 2014), 32.

108. Elizabeth Lipski, *Digestive Wellness: Strengthen the Immune System and Prevent Disease Through Healthy Digestion,* 4th ed. (New York, NY: McGraw-Hill Education, 2011), 247.

109. Elizabeth Lipski, *Digestive Wellness: Strengthen the Immune System and Prevent Disease Through Healthy Digestion,* 4th ed. (New York, NY: McGraw-Hill Education, 2011), 247.

110. American Institute for Cancer Research, *The AICR Guide to the Nutrition Facts Label*. (Washington, DC. AICR Publications), E2A-NF, 1

111. AICR Healthy Recipes. http://www.aicr.org/can-prevent/healthy-recipes/.

112. Gary Taubes, *Good Calories, Bad Calories,* (lecture, Institute for Integrative Nutrition, Health coach Training Curriculum course, module 21, September 2014).

113. Lyle MacWilliam, *NutriSearch Comparative Guide to Nutritional Supplements,* 5th ed. (Kelowna, BC: Northern Dimensions Publishing, 2014), 13-18.

114. Ron Kennedy, "Short History of Vitamins," The Doctors' Medical Library, (accessed March 2018), 3. http://www.medical-library.net/short-history-of-vitamins/

115. Ron Kennedy, "Short History of Vitamins," The Doctors' Medical Library, (accessed March 2018), 1. http://www.medical-library.net/short-history-of-vitamins/

116. "Dietary Supplements-Food and Drug Administration," FDA publishers. (accessed June 2018), 1. https://www.fda.gov/Food/DietarySupplement/

117. "Dietary Supplements: What You Need To Know," FDA publishers. (accessed June 2018), 3. https://www.fda.gov/Food/DietarySupplement/UsingDietarySupplements/default.htm.

118. "Dietary Supplements-Food and Drug Administration," FDA publishers. (accessed June 2018),1. https://www.fda.gov/Food/DietarySupplement/.

119. Lyle MacWilliam, *NutriSearch Comparative Guide to Nutritional Supplements,* 5th ed. (Kelowna, BC: Northern Dimensions Publishing, 2014), 13.

120. "Independent tests and reviews of vitamin, minerals" Consumer Lab.Com Publishers, (accessed June 2018), https://www.consumerlab.com/Independent tests and reviews of vitamin, mineral....

121. Lyle MacWilliam, *NutriSearch Comparative Guide to Nutritional Supplements,* 5th ed. (Kelowna, BC: Northern Dimensions Publishing, 2014), https://www.Nutrisearch.ca

122. "Recommended Daily intakes and Upper Limits for Nutrients" Consumer Lab.Com Publishers, (accessed June 2018), https://www.consumerlab.com/RDAs

123. Lyle MacWilliam, *NutriSearch Comparative Guide to Nutritional Supplements,* 5th ed. (Kelowna, BC: Northern Dimensions Publishing, 2014), 7.

124. Lyle MacWilliam, *utriSearch Comparative Guide to Nutritional Supplements,* 5th ed. (Kelowna, BC: Northern Dimensions Publishing, 2014), 27.

125. Lyle MacWilliam, *utriSearch Comparative Guide to Nutritional Supplements,* 5th ed. (Kelowna, BC: Northern Dimensions Publishing, 2014), 44.

126. Joshua Rosenthal, *Integrative Nutrition: Feed Your Hunger for Health & Happiness,* 3rd ed. (New York, NY: Integrative Nutrition Publishing, 2014), 168–171.

127. Joshua Rosenthal, I*Integrative Nutrition: Feed Your Hunger for Health & Happiness,* 3rd ed. (New York, NY: Integrative Nutrition Publishing, 2014), 191.

128. Joshua Rosenthal, "The Circle of Life," (lecture, Institute for Integrative Nutrition, Health Coach Training Curriculum course, Module 3, The Circle of Life, September 2013), 2.

129. Abraham Verghese, "Spirituality and Mental Health," *Indian Journal of Psychiatry* 50 no.4 (October–December 2008): 233–237.

130. Joshua Rosenthal, *Integrative Nutrition: Feed Your Hunger for Health & Happiness,* 3rd ed. New York, NY: Integrative Nutrition Publishing, 2014), 190.

131. Joshua Rosenthal, "The Circle of Life," (lecture, Institute for Integrative Nutrition, Health Coach Training Curriculum course, Module 3, The Circle of Life, September 2013), 2.

132. Elizabeth Lipski, *Digestive Wellness: Strengthen the Immune System and Prevent Disease Through Healthy Digestion,* 4th ed. (New York, NY: McGraw-Hill Education, 2011), 133.

133. Arne Garborg, *IZQuotes, Authors, Writers, Celebrities,* http://izquotes.com/authors/ quote/343063

134. American Institute for Cancer Research, *Move More to Reduce Your Cancer Risk.* (Washington, DC: AICR Publications, E51-MM, November 2004, 8.

135. "Work out benefits" accessed 2014, http;//www.consumerreports.org/health/free-highlights/manage-your-health/workout-benefits.htm.

136. American Institute for Cancer Research, *Move More to Reduce Your Cancer Risk*. (Washington, DC: AICR Publications, E51-MM, November 2004). 13.

137. Experience Life Staff, "The Calorie Myth," *Experience Life,* September 2014, https://experiencelife.com/article/the-calorie-myth/.

138. Experience Life Staff, "The Calorie Myth," *Experience Life,* September 2014, https://experiencelife.com/article/the-calorie-myth/.

139. Experience Life Staff, "The Calorie Myth," *Experience Life,* September 2014, https://experiencelife.com/article/the-calorie-myth/.

140. Experience Life Staff, "The Calorie Myth," *Experience Life,* September 2014, https://experiencelife.com/article/the-calorie-myth/.

141. Experience Life Staff, "The Calorie Myth," *Experience Life,*, September 2014, https://experiencelife.com/article/the-calorie-myth/.

142. Phil Mutz, "12 Incredible Ways To Add Joy To Your Life," Little Things, accessed June 2018. https://www.littlethings.com/easy-ways-to-add-joy-to-your-life/.

143. Phil Mutz, "12 Incredible Ways To Add Joy To Your Life," Little Things, accessed June 2018. https://www.littlethings.com/easy-ways-to-add-joy-to-your-life/.

144. American Institute for Cancer Research, *The New American Plate: Meals For A Healthy Weight and A Healthy Life*. (Washington, DC. AICR Publications, E4B-NAP revised November 2014). 5.

145. "Food Combining Simplified," (Institute for Integrative Nutrition, Health Coach Training Curriculum course, module 13, 2013).

146. American Institute for Cancer Research, *Moving Toward a Plant-Based Diet: Menus and Recipes for Cancer Prevention Healthy Living and Lower Cancer Risk* (Washington, DC. AICR Publications, November 2001), E1B-PBD/F41, 2.

147. Annemarie Colbin, *Food and Healing: How What You Eat Determines Your Health, Your Well-Being, and the Quality of Your Life,* 10th ed. (New York, NY: Ballantine Books, 1986), 75.

148. Lyle MacWilliam, *NutriSearch Comparative Guide to Nutritional Supplements,* 5th ed. (Kelowna, BC: Northern Dimensions Publishing, 2014), 10.

149. Experience Life Staff, "Why Healthy Humans Need Healthy Soil, *Conventional – Farming Practices That Harm the Soil,*" Experience Life, April 2017, https://experiencelife.com/article/got-soil-why-healthy-humans-need-healthy-soil/.

150. "EWG's 2017 Shopper's Guide to Pesticides in Produce," Executive Summary, Environmental Working Group, accessed April 2018. https://www.ewg.org/foodnews/summary.php

151. "EWG's 2017 Shopper's Guide to Pesticides in Produce," Executive Summary, Environmental Working Group, accessed April 2018. https://www.ewg.org/foodnews/summary.php

152. "Fruits, Veggies and Pesticides," (lecture, Joshua Rosenthal, Institute for Integrative Nutrition, Health Coach Training Curriculum course of 2013, module 19, February 2014).

153. "The Great Organic Debate Get to Know Your PLU'S," (lecture, Joshua Rosenthal, Institute for Integrative Nutrition, Health Coach Training Curriculum course of 2013, module 19, February 2014).

154. American Institute for Cancer Research, *The New American Plate: Meals For A Healthy Weight and A Healthy Life.* (Washington, DC. AICR Publications, E4B-NAP revised November 2014). 5.

155. "Food Combining Simplified," (lecture, Joshua Rosenthal, Institute for Integrative Nutrition, Health Coach Training Curriculum course of 2013, module 13, December 2013).

156. "Food Combining Simplified," (lecture, Joshua Rosenthal, Institute for Integrative Nutrition, Health Coach Training Curriculum course of 2013, module 13, December 2013).

157. Institute for Integrative Nutrition®, *Portion Size,* Handout (New York, NY: Institute for Integrative Nutrition®, September 2013).

158. Susan Smith Jones, *Herbs: Nature's Medicine Chest* (Sherman Oaks, CA: Health Point Press, 2010) 2.

159. Dr. Seuss, *"Oh, The Places You'll Go!"* (London: Harper Collins, 2003), 42.

Made in the USA
Monee, IL
09 November 2019